GETTING

WELL

Contents: What is Health; The Rationale of Disease;
Compensation in Disease; Law Governs Disease;
Physiology vs. Voodooism; The Story of Useless Organs;
The Fun of Being Sick; How to get Well; Why Drugs;
Quick Relief; Killing our Children; Curing Arthritis;
Peptic Ulcers; What are Tumors; Curing Gallstones;
Diabetes; Varicose Veins; Asthma; Warts; Influenza;
Who's on a A Diet; Food cures; Vitamin Failures; When
to Eat; Growing Old; Diseases of Middle Life; plus more.

Herbert M. Shelton

ISBN 1-56459-980-9

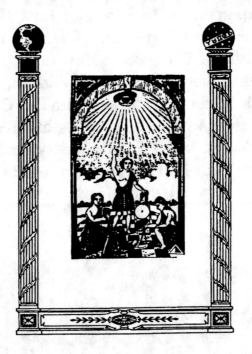

Kessinger Publishing Company
Montana, U.S.A.

Warning—Disclaimer

This book is intended as a historical reference volume only, not as a medical guide or a manual for self-treatment.

The information presented herein is in no way intended as a substitute for medical counseling or for any treatment prescribed by your doctor. The information given is not medical advice nor is it presented as medical advice. It is not intended to diagnose or treat an individual's health problem or ailments.

It is sold with the understanding that the publisher and the author are not liable for the misconception or misuse of any information provided. The Publisher shall have neither liability nor responsibility to any person or entity with respect to any loss, damage, or injury caused or alleged to be caused directly or indirectly by the information contained in this book.

If you suspect that you have a medical problem, please seek competent medical care.

Far too large a section of the treatment of disease is today controlled by the big manufacturing pharmacists, who have enslaved us in a plausible pseudo-science.

Sir Wm. Osler, in *Oxford Medicine*

INDEX

The disgrace of medicine has been that colossal system of self-deception, in obedience to which mines have been emptied of their cankering minerals, the entrals of animals taken for their impurities, the poison bags of reptiles drained of their venom, and all the inconceivable absurdities thus obtained thrust down the throats of human beings suffering from some want of organization, nourishment or vital stimulation.

—Dr. Oliver Wendell Holmes

Introduction

This is a day of sensational discoveries and miracle medicines. Remarkable new cures and near-panceas are of frequent discovery. Snake venom, artificial fever, frozen sleep, the sulfonamides, penicillin, streptothricin, blood plasma, more powerful X-rays — these vie with sports and movies for free newspaper space. So much is claimed for them and so many new discoveries are made in relation to them that the public is kept constantly keyed up with open-mouthed and wild-eyed expectancy.

At long last, "science" is staging a powerful and winning Blitz-Krieg against man's ancient and implacable foe — *disease*. With remarkable and sensational discoveries crowding so closely one upon the heels of another, the time is surely not far distant when universal health will prevail.

Not only is ours an age of remarkable cures, it is also a time of equally remarkable preventives. We now have so many "successful" vaccines and serums, that there is no longer any need for anyone ever to suffer from many of the "diseases" that were so common yesteryear. New serums are of frequent discovery so that we may look forward hopefully to the time when all "disease" will be conquered.

Surgery, too, has made rapid strides. It has grown more daring and is, today, invading physiological precincts, which only a few years ago, it would not have dared touch. With the newer advances in surgery added to the new cures and the new serums and vaccines we have an almost ideal combination for the "conquest of disease."

What these three groups of anti-disease weapons lack in power and effectiveness is completely made up by the many glandular products (hormones) and vitamin combinations that are claimed to do so much for the sick. There is, surely, no longer reason to doubt that the *Golden Age* has arrived.

The intelligent and informed reader, however, will notice one very important defect in all of these methods of cure and prevention. He will quickly detect a deficiency for which no amount of shouting can compensate. It is this:

None of these methods of cure and prevention are designed to affect or even touch the real, the basic, cause of disease .

Drugs may suppress symptoms but they do not remove cause. They may kill germs (they also kill patients), but they do not clear up the systemic condition that permits germs to thrive and grow in the body. "Frozen sleep" may tempararily check the growth of a tumor or cancer, but it does not and cannot remove the cause of cancer. Radium or powerful X-rays may destroy a cancerous growth but they do not and cannot remove the cause of cancer. It must be emphasized that

If it does not remove cause, it does not cure.

Serums and vaccines are admittedly capable of doing much harm, but they do not prevent the cause of disease. They do not enable us to avoid the cause of disease. We need to know that

If they do not enable us to avoid the cause of disease they do not prevent disease.

Surgery may pull a tooth, extract the tonsils, remove the gall-bladder, excise the appendix, cut out the ovaries or the seminal vesicles, drain the sinuses, etc., but it cannot remove the cause of disease. It is time for us to understand that

INTRODUCTION

If surgery does not remove the cause of disease, it does not cure.

There is no cure short of removal of cause. Cutting out an organ, suppressing a symptom, destroying a growth, removing a stone — these processes touch effects only. They fail to restore health for three very vital reasons:

1. They do not remove the cause of ill-health.

2. They are not the factors out of which good health is built.

3. They produce positive injury of the body.

For prevention of "disease" and recovery of health we must look to constructive natural agents, forces and methods and cease relying on destructive, unnatural or anti-natural measures, agents and processes. Agents that produce disease in the well are not well adapted to the production of health in the sick. Disease-producing agents and measures are not health-preserving. The popular methods of prevention and *cure* neither prevent nor cure. Witness the evergrowing army of sick and suffering in spite of the ever-increasing size of our army of physicians, the ever-increasing number and size of our hospitals and the ever-growing list of cures and preventives.

To avoid sickness, avoid the cause of sickness. Only madness can lead us to attempt to prevent disease by producing disease.

To "cure" disease, remove the causes of disease. It would be the worst kind of folly to attempt to cure disease by ignoring its causes and employing other causes of disease.

To build health, employ the cause of health. How foolish to attempt to build health by employing means that are known to impair and wreck health.

In the following pages the causes of disease and the ways of health are made plain. Not mehods of *cure*, but a plan of living is there presented for those who can understand.

For twenty-six years the author of this little book, the contents of which first appeared as magazine articles in *Dr. Shelton's Hygienic Review*, has been leading the sick back to health and teaching the well how to remain so. For eighteen years *Dr. Shelton's Health School* has been employing the health building means described in these pages. While at the *Health School* we have received a great preponderance of scraps and derelicts, those who have suffered for years and "have tried everything" without avail, our success in building good health in the great majority of these sufferers has been remarkable.

At the *Health School* we have no cure-all, in fact, we have no *cure* at all. We recognize that only nature (meaning the forces and processes of life) can cure and we accord to nature the opportunity as well as the power of cure. Ours is a plan of living and a program of education. If this seems too simple, if it is not mysterious enough, if it seems to lack power, just think over this fact:

If this plan were ineffectual we could not succeed where all others fail.

Of the reader we ask only an intelligent hearing. Lay aside your prejudices and prepossessions and do some real honest-to-goodness thinking as you read the pages of this little book. Then, when you thoroughly understand its contents, give them a fair and honest test. Heed the ancient admonition: "Prove (test) all things, hold fast that which is good" (true).

An old adage has it that "the proof of the pudding is in the eating thereof." The proof of the truth of the principles presented in this book and of the value of the practices built thereon is in making use of them. "The wise will understand."

What Is Health?

Efforts to define health have not given very satisfactory results. The dictionary defines health as a "state of bodily or mental well being; normal condition of mind or body in which all parts and faculties perform their functions duly, easily, satisfactorily; soundness, freedom from disease, disorder, pain or weakness."

The word is from the anglo-saxon and means wholeness, integrity. It is thought that originally the word had reference to the absence of obvious bodily wounds and injuries and had little or no reference to the deeper and more obscure processes of life. Be this as it may, wholeness is no mere negative thing — it is not the mere absence of loss. It is a positive thing and signifies the presence of parts and functions. To define it as "freedom from weakness and disease" is to define it in a very negative manner and to rob it of the most essential part of its meaning. To say that health is the absence of disease is merely to say that health is the absence of discomfort — or, it is a state of comfort. This covers but a small part of health.

Pathologists, we are told, have long felt the need for a definition of health in terms of resistance to disease. Such a definition would be a fallacy. There is no such thing —entity— as disease to resist. The whole concept of *resistance* with reference to disease is based on a very ancient and very wrong conception of the nature of the process called disease. There are many things to resist, but disease is not one of them. Any definition of health that does not include more positive factors than that of the mere idea of *resistance to disease* must fail to properly define it.

Health must be defined in terms of biological and physiological efficiency and integrity. Any definition of health that regards the individual as an isolated unit and fails to consider his functions in nature must fall short of a complete definition.

Prof. J. Arthur Thompson says that the body is now regarded as a chemical and physical system and that "by health we mean mainly useful, efficient, and harmonious production of energy." He asserts that this production of energy depends more upon general functional harmony and perfection than upon structural integrity.

Up to the time of his death Prof. Thomson was the British chief priest of the cult of Darwinism and as a Darwinian he was unwilling to recognize the pathological condition of all forms of life that have strayed from the path of biological rectitude and, as a consequence, have undergone degeneration ("simplification" in Darwinian language) and acromegaly ("over-specialization", the Darwinians call it.) Pathology of a whole species, even of the whole genera, is health in his language.

The body does not merely produce energy, it also expends energy. It works. It also reproduces. Health involves not only the ability to produce energy, but also the ability to use it and the ability to reproduce. Loss of structure or impairment of structure means loss of ability to work. It should also be said that pathological reproduction is common in nature.

We cannot accept Thompson's definition of health nor his negation of the importance of structural integrity. Unless he or some of his echoes, can show us that function (we will not ask for "general functional harmony and perfection") can go on in a vacuum, we will continue to believe that structural integrity is essential to "general functional harmony and perfection." Function without structure simply does not exist.

He tells us that if a man's temperature is normal, his heart sound, his blood pure and of good quality and if there are no microbes in his veins, "even if the man has lost an arm or a leg or an eye, we can label him healthy, and can safely infer that he has normal health, i.e. normal capacity for work."

For what kind of work does a one-eyed man possess normal capacity? For what kind of work does the one-armed or one-legged man possess normal capacity? Work must not mean merely the various artificial occupations of civilization. We must not exclude or neglect biological work.

He makes the same kind of mistake when he says: "There is no great advantage in the possession of large muscles and great muscular energy.* * * Perfect health is possible without unusual muscular devlopment, muscular strength, or muscular endurance."

We presume that the parasite that has lost eyes, head, feet, wings, and digestive system would, if it could talk, also say that perfect health is possible without the possession of these things. At least the parasite can "survive" without these organs and parts and "survival" is the all-important thing in Prof. Thompson's view.

Muscles are part of the body; indeed they form a great part of it and any statement that perfect health is possible when these are in a state of neglect or under-development, is ridiculous. The organic correlations and interdependencies within the body make it necessary that full health involves muscular development.

—11—

Change of structure is not altogether a local affair, but carries with it certain consequences in the nature of correlated changes in other parts of the body. These correlated changes are also functional and not merely structural. Relations and correlations depend upon function and when function is impaired or suspended, every relation and correlation is correspondingly limited.

The removal of relatively "unimportant" organs may be rashly declared to result in no harm; an individual who is a veritable caricature of a human being due to antithetic development, may be as rashly declared to be healthy, but such foolish declarations ignore functional and structural relations and correlations. How foolish to declare the eunuch or the spayed woman to be healthy and all the while ignore all the results of the surgical spoilation of these people. Internal physiological stability is a prerequisite to efficiency of external biological function. Asymmetry, disharmony, antithetic developments, dwarfism, giantism, acromegaly and all other departures from the norms of life are pathological and their possessor is not healthy. It will not do to declare, as Professor Thompson does, that disease is relative and undefinable. If we fail to adequately define the abnormal, we are not, thereby, justified in including it in the category of normal.

Harry Benjamin, a British Natural Therapist, writing in the July (1943) issue of *Health for All*, attempts to define health for us. He rightly points out that what the medical profession and the average individual means by health is only *average health*. He says that what passes for a healthy man or woman today is someone who may have defective teeth, impaired vision, flat feet, faulty body posture, and minor ailments such as constipation and catarrh. Mr. Average man and woman do not know what health really is and adopt a definition that would fit Prof. Thomson's conceptions.

Dr. Benjamin also falls into this same trap. He declares that health "has nothing to do with extra muscular development, or with strength in the sense of purely physical strength • • • . Whether that body be very muscular and physically strong does not enter into the matter. If all the organs of the body are working efficiently, it must mean that the muscular system is properly developed throughout the body. Excessive muscular development does not mean an extra degree of health."

His last statement is empty of all meaning for the reason that he does not define "excessive muscular development." But it does seem strange to us that a man can recognize poor vision as an evidence of poor health and then claim that muscular condition is relatively unimportant to health. He seems to think a state of comparative muscular weakness is compatible with a high degree of health.

He is not consistent, however, for he does unconsciously recognize the correlation of health and muscular condition when he says that if all the organs of the body are working efficiently it must mean that the muscles are properly developed throughout the body. If it can be shown that the muscles are not properly developed throughout, it must follow that all the organs of the body are not working efficiently.

Dr. Benjamin falls into his errors because he adopts a very narrow and onesided definition of health. Although he insists that health is different from the condition of "just not being unwell," he describes it as "a feeling of 'alivenes,' a feeling of bouyancy and ease in movements, and a zest in work and activity; and with it goes a readiness to face life and its problems and not shirk them or pass them on to other peoples' shoulders." • • • it is just a *feeling* pure and simple; a feeling which comes from within, owing to the natural and easy functions of all the organs, glands and other vital machinery of life."

This effort to define health as *feeling* is as wrong as Prof. Thompson's effort to define it as ability to produce energy. Zestfulness and a feeling of ease and aliveness go with health, but they are not health. They are expressions of health.

Health is biological as well as physiological and is based on biological as well as upon physiological factors. It is a state of wholeness — of structural integrity and functional efficiency— based on hygienic living and wholesome biological relations. It does not matter how good one·feels today, if his relations and conduct are not what they should be, he will not feel so good tomorrow. It does not matter how efficiently he produces energy today, if his conduct and relations flout the laws of life, his energy production will fag tomorrow. If he is not whole, entire, he cannot have perfect health or even near-perfect health. The half-man can never have the health of the whole-man.

The Rationale of Disease

Against their own wills, physiologists were driven to a recognition of what certain ancients called the "law of the members." Indeed, the interdependence of the organs of the body has aroused the wonderment of physiologists. No longer is it considered the legitimate function of science to isolate the parts and treat them as though they had a separate existence of their own. It is now the effort of science to get a clear picture of the *tout ensemble*. The mere specialist's view is, in the long run, inadequate and unsatisfactory.

Physiologists have been forced to the conclusion that what happens at one place in the body is in consonance with what is occurring at another. In fact, it is now well known that every part acts more distinctly for the good of the whole than for its own advantage.

It remains only that this same principle be recognized in the workings of the body in "disease" for the science of physiology to be complete. The time has come when it is necessary for us to cease thinking of what is called "morbid function" as outside of or apart from physiology.

We have also to cease thinking of this so-called "morbid function" as, of itself, an evil. How can we consistently hold that inflammation is both a constructive, a healing, process and, at the same time, an evil? How can we hold that fever is both curative and destructive?

The behaviour of the body in those states called *disease* represents mere modifications—for the most part, exaggerations or diminutions — of its ordinary or normal behavior. They are as truly vital or physiological as the ordinary activities of life.

If we can learn to see them, not only as modifications of the ordinary activities of life, but as modifications that are made to serve definite and useful ends, we can get away from the ancient, though still prevailing, conception of "disease" as an *attack* upon the body by some outside force or entity. We can see that, apart from the body itself, disease has no existence.

Disease does not attack us. It is, rather, the name we have given to the processes by which we attack the foes of life. We do not resist disease. Disease is part of the process by which we resist the foes of life. When we vomit a poison that has been swallowed, this process is part of our resistance to the poison. If the drug is expelled by means of a diarrhea this is only another means we have of resisting the poison.

There is as much sense in calling the processes by which we resist and expel poisons, evil, as there would be in calling the process of tanning, by which we resist an excess of the sun's rays, an evil.

I can see no objection to distinguishing between the two sets of actions — the ordinary or *normal* process of living and the extraordinary or *abnormal* process of living — for convenience of study, but only so long as this is not allowed to obscure their fundamental oneness or identity.

The difference between a diarrhea and a normal bowel action is one of degree, not of kind. It is wrong to attribute normal *bowel* action to the powers of life (call it physiological) and then attribute the abnormal bowel action to some attacking force (call it non-physiological). The action in both instances is the same. In both instances, too, it serves the same purpose — namely, the expulsion of unwanted or injurious materials.

In speaking of the cause of disease, it is well for us to have a clear understanding of what we mean by disease. Fever is caused by the same powers of life that produce *normal* body temperature. Inflammation is caused by the same powers of life that cause *normal* circulation. Diarrhea is caused by the same physiological powers that cause *normal* bowel action.

All vital or physiological actions, whether called *normal* or *abnormal*, are caused by the same vital or physiological powers. Outside forces do not cause the actions of the body. The cause of vital actions is resident in the living organism.

Poisons — toxins — cause injury, not physiological or vital processes and actions. The injury or threat of injury is the *occasion* for action, not the cause of the action.

If poisons could cause action, there seems to be no reason why a strong purgative could not cause action in the bowels of the dead. But the cause of action is elsewhere and when that cause of action is gone, no action follows no matter what is done to induce it.

It is one thing to produce damage — it is another thing to produce function, even modified function. What we are to regard as the cause of *disease* must depend upon which of the three separate sets or groups of phenomena commonly included under this generic term we mean by disease.

Cut a man with a knife. We have:

(1) The act of cutting and the agent of cutting — the knife.

(2) The cut.

(3) The pain, bleeding, inflammation and other vital phenomena that follow at the site of the cut.

The knife causes the cut, it does not cause the inflammation. In current literature of disease we have all three of the above sets of facts called disease.

The vital actions — defensive, reparative, eliminative, recuperative — are called disease.

The condition of injury produced by poisons, toxins, parasites, fire, cold, etc., is called disease.

The cause of the injury is called disease.

Take your choice.

Until these three groups of distinct phenomena are carefully separated, both in our minds and in our terminology, there is no hope of escape from the present almost universal confusion about a subject that should be simple and easily understood.

Compensation in Disease

Compensation is a balancing of accounts. It is to weigh together or counterbalance. The principle of compensation seems to be universal in its application. Perhaps if we could all fully realize this important fact we would stop many practices we now carry on, end many institutions we now support, give up many beliefs we now hold, and cease many strivings we now make.

That many ancient people had a deep insight into the working of the principle of compensation is shown by aphorisms that they have handed down to us. "As ye give, so shall ye receive"; "Whatsoever a man soweth, that shall he also reap."; "Let him that would be greatest among you be the least among you."; "The rewards of life are for service, its penalties for self-indulgence."; "We derive our greatest happiness from making others happy," are only a few evidences of the recognition of the principle of compensation, or of service and counter-service.

The principle of compensation is seen in biology, not merely in the rewards and penalties meted out to organisms for (or by) their good or bad conduct (whether service or depradation), but also in the developments of their very bodies. Darwin was so blinded by his pet hypothesis of "natural selection" that he consigned compensation to the sphere of physiology where it has, since that time, led a charmed life. Darwin called the principle of compensation "balancement of growth."

He was of the opinion that the principle of compensation "holds true to a certain extent with our domestic productions: if nourishment flows to one part or another in excess, it rarely flows, at least in excess, to another part; thus it is difficult to get a cow to give milk and to fatten readily. The same varieties of the cabbage do not yield abundant and nutritious foliage and a copious supply of oil-bearing seeds. When the seeds in our fruits become atrophied, the fruit itself gains largely in size and quality. In our poultry, a large tuft of feathers on the head is usually accompanied by a diminished comb, and a large beard by diminished wattles."

Although admitting that "many good observers, more especially botanists," believed to the contrary, Darwin adds: "with species in a state of nature, it can hardly be maintained that the law is of universal application." He seems to have regarded compensation as a merely casual phenomenon, occurring occasionally in the physiological economy of the organism. Perhaps this was due to his inability to fit it into parson Malthus' struggle for existence.

Goethe expressed the law of compensation thus: "in order to spend on the one side, Nature is forced to economize on the other side." It would be possible to fill several volumes with examples of this fact, but we lack time and space for the work and are at present, at least, chiefly interested in the application of the principle to the phenomena of disease.

To save in one department as against special expenditure in another is a fundamental necessity of organic life. A few examples must suffice. If one is attempting to solve an intricate problem in mathematics he must give his whole and undivided attention (this is called concentration) to the work. It would be impossible for him to work even simple mathematical problems and run at top speed at the same time. The old Roman proverb, "a full stomach does not like to think," expresses the fact that the digestion of a meal detracts from mental powers. Hyperemia (excess of blood) in one part of the body produces by way of compensation, a deficiency of blood (anemia) in another part. The flow of energy, like the flow of blood, to parts of the body is governed by the same law of compensation.

The organs of the body are not independent isonomies. They are parts of a unified and correlated organism. Every organ depends upon every other organ. What an organ may spend depends upon the adequacy of support it receives from the other organs; that is, it depends upon compensation. If an organ becomes wasteful of the funds of life, it weakens not only itself, but the body as a whole.

If sexual excesses deplete the powers of life they do not merely produce sexual impotence, they weaken and exhaust the whole body. If gluttony is allowed to waste the funds of the organism, this does not stop with the weakening of the digestive system. The whole body is weakened. Organs that cease to serve and that merely indulge steal from themselves at the same time they steal from the body.

The funds of life are limited. There are people whose reckless indulgence would lead us to think that they doubt this simple fact. There are symptom-treaters who so waste the powers of their patients and defend their enervating practices, that we naturally conclude that they also think the funds of life are inexhaustible.

The limited funds of life plus the fact that expenditure depends on compensation, render it impossible that all, or many, parts of the organism can simultaneously receive excessive supplies or even that one part can receive a great excess and all others receive normal supplies. "In order to spend on one side, Nature is forced to economize on the other side."

In the enervated organism that has become so toxemic and, perhaps, so infected, that a crisis is produced, the limited forces of the depleted organism must be mobilized for the immediate task of preventing damage and saving life. Great and unusual expenditure is called for in a new direction and this at a time when the funds of life are below normal.

The demand for funds can be met only by great and unusual reductions of activities in other and normal directions. Prostration, which means that the sick person becomes so weak physically, that he is "floored" or put to bed, represents an "economizing on the other side." It means that the funds regularly expended in physical activities are now available for expenditure in the temporarily more important work of elimination, defense and healing. Suspension of the digestive processes represents the same compensatory adjustment. The energy and blood regularly used in digesting and absorbing the daily food is now withdrawn from these channels and turned into other and temporarily more important channels. Thus relieved of some of its burdens, the organism is able to make new exertions in other directions and to progress accordingly.

This re-cannalization of the body's energies and funds is automatic and directed from within. It takes place in strictest conformity with the laws of life and no mistakes are made. For this reason among others, it is always dangerous for the symptom-treater to attempt to interfere with the orderly course of disease — to suppress activity where nature has increased it and to excite increased activity where she has decreased or suspended it. Treating symptoms is always a slap at compensation.

Practitioners who are addicted to any of the stimulating practices (drug or drugless) in vogue should be made to realize that there is no such thing as perpetual motion to be had out of an organ or an organism. This kind of exploitation of the funds of life leads inevitably to morbidity and degeneracy.

Normally, compensation is very precise, but it is only on a *tout-ensemble* view of the organism that we can see the principle in its proper setting. The average practitioner, unfortunately, tends to isolate the parts of the body and treat them as though they led separate and independent existences.

The organs of the body are co-equal partners in a vital reciprocity. They work together for the common good. Some work while others receive. Some rest while others work. Some abstain while others are supplied. Those in receipt of extra supplies are to use them for extra services to their physiological partners. The universal truth is that where pronounced activity is required from an organ or from a physiologic system, this may be obtained provided the organism possesses sufficient funds to pay for the extra work.

When man consciously intervenes in this process he tends to disarrange the vital adjustments that have been made. He obtains the coveted extra activity in an inhibited organ at the expense of funds badly needed elsewhere. He inhibits "over-active" organs at the cost of reducing their curative work. In either case, greater weakness results. His actions resemble those of the bull in the China shop.

The symptom-treater cannot thus interfere with the activities of an organ or system without at the same time, and as a direct consequence, alter the relations and correlations of those activities. Every other activity or modification of activity in the·body that depends, either directly or indirectly, upon the increased or decreased activity of the organ he treats, is interfered with commensurate with his interference with their support. For example, if he reduces temperature, every modification of function in the whole body that depends upon the fever, will be, accordingly, suppressed.

If modification of function is, *per se*, an evil, this suppressive work might be justified. For example, if the excess of blood sent to the tissues around a wound is an evil, if it is not essential to protection and healing, it might be well to suppress the inflammation. But if the excess of blood serves a useful, a necessary, purpose, what but evil can flow from its suppression?

Compensation does not miss us when·we resort to therapeutic devices to "cure" our "diseases." We are forced to pay in increased and prolonged suffering, greater weakness, even by death, for our meddlesome interference with the processes of life as these are altered or modified to meet the varying conditions and circumstances of life.

Law Governs Disease

If the principles of development hold good in the normal or healthy states of organisms, they ought, surely, to apply equally to diseased conditions. Facts clearly indicate that "disease" is controlled by the same laws which regulate biological processes in general. "Disease," being controlled by natural conditions, cannot be regarded as unnatural. We must not confuse *unnatural* with *abnormal*.

"Disease," in many instances, may be regarded as exaggerated function so that the manifestations of disease are regulated by the same laws which govern physiological processes in general. Functions may not only be exaggerated, they may also be diminished. A man may not only run at top speed, he may also lay down and sleep.

Functions may be greatly increased in one direction and, by way of compensation, be equally reduced in another. Not only are functions increased or decreased, but structures also undergo similar modifications. If exercise will cause a development of larger and stronger muscles, lack of exercise will cause them to grow smaller and weaker. Compensation is ever and forever in the balance — well or sick, the law of compensation never deserts its post. Let us observe a few examples and see what important lesson we can draw from them.

It is generally believed that the loss of one eye causes the vision of the other eye to improve. Although often denied, this is probably correct. It is asserted by good authority that when an eye is lost in early life, the other eye "aquires a greater range of movement and quickness which compensates in no small degree for the loss of its companion." It is also claimed that in persons blind from early life, the power of hearing becomes wonderfully quickened. The sense of hearing of the mole is proverbial. "Pray you tread softly that the blind mole may not hear a footfall," says Caliban to Stephano in *Trinculo*. The blind fish in the mammoth cave are said to be "abnormally sensitive" to sounds. Need I point out that the added work thrown upon one arm by the loss of the other results in increased size and efficiency of the remaining arm?

When an organ is called upon to do more work, it is strengthened for this purpose. This is the secret of muscular development through exercise. It is the secret of "wind" and endurance through running. It is the secret of improving vision by using the eyes, of cultivating acute perception of minute differences in sounds seen in musicians.

The above examples of enlargement of parts and increased abilities of parts to compensate for loss of parts and the enlargement and strengthening of parts to meet increased demands, may be regarded as belonging to the young. It may be thought that no compensation of this kind can occur in older people.

While it is true that the process is seen in its greatest perfection in the young and we would hardly expect to see any enlargement of the bones in a man past fifty to give greater strength, were he to begin carrying heavy loads, yet it is a fact that compensating processes, both of a structural and functional nature, are seen in older men and women.

Enlargement of parts to compensate for the loss of other parts may be seen in old people. There is the classic example of the loss of her big toe by a woman of fifty. Six months after she regained the use of her foot, the second toe had enlarged and stood out from its fellows to such an extent that it bore such striking resemblance in size and general appearance to the big toe, that when the foot was exhibited to a class of students, the large second toe was mistaken for the hallus or big toe. The increase in the size and strength of this toe was made necessary by the increased work it was forced to do after the loss of the big toe.

It is well known that the loss of one kidney is followed by the enlargement of the remaining kidney; thus compensating for the loss and saving the owner from disaster. This compensating enlargement of a kidney has been seen most often in man following removal of one kidney, but it has also been observed in horses, cows, sheep, pheasants, hens and, perhaps, other animals.

Organs thus increased in size are said to be hypertrophied. It arises in the kidney, as in the above mentioned case of the increase size of the second toe, to meet increased demands upon it. Although hypertropy in both of these conditions is regarded as *pathological* because it arises under abnormal conditions, whereas hypertrophy arising under normal conditions, is regarded as functional, it will be seen that both forms of hypertrophy are the same, are controlled by identical laws and represent responses to similar demands for increased function of the part.

We may say, then, that *hypertrophy* is any increase in size above the optimum normal size of an organ to provide for increased function demanded of the part. "Enlargement of a part from such cause is said to be compensatory." Instead, then, of *hypertrophy* being, *per se*, an evil, it is an effort to offset or counterbalance an evil.

Enlargement of the tonsils is a familiar case of hypertrophy. In the case of the tonsils, the enlargement is not permanent because the need for the enlargement is not permanent. It may be permissible to say that *hypertrophy* may be either temporary or permanent depending on the need that called it into existence.

Enlargement of the tonsils is due to the same thing that occasions enlargement of one kidney when the other is removed. In the case of the kidneys, when one is removed, the remaining kidney is called upon to remove the waste that they both formerly removed. In other words, it has twice as much work to do. The only way in which it can do twice as much work is by enlarging, thus increasing its working capacity.

In toxic states, the tonsils, which are parts of the body's toxin-destroying system, are often forced to enlarge because the toxic load is too great for them to handle at their normal size. They, thus, hypertrophy for the same reason that the kidney does—to increase their working capacity.

When the toxic state has been reduced and the extra work is no longer required of the tonsils, they return to their normal size. There is no way of supplying the body with another kidney, so that the extra work thrown upon the remaining one is a permanent job. The *hypertrophy* in its case is also permanent.

Numerous examples of both temporary and permanent variations in the size of a part according to the work it performs are seen throughout nature. Not all forms of overgrowth fall into this classification. There are overgrowths due to diminished use and overgrowths due to prolonged irritation. Of this latter, tumors are a common example.

Irritation results in overgrowth in much the same way that increased use does. Additional blood is sent to points of irritation just as it is sent to parts that are used. If the irritation is chronic the additional blood to the part is also chronic and this results in overgrowth. Corns and callouses are also familiar examples of overgrowth due to irritation. At least, in these two cases, the thickening and overgrowth of the skin is definitely protective.

Hooves, spurs, claws, beaks, nails, etc., that grow throughout life to compensate for the constant wear to which they are subjected by use, tend to grow larger or longer or both, when not used. ·

Study of the enlargement of parts arising from increased use, diminished use, additional blood supply, and irritation, shows clearly enough that the same laws which regulate these processes under normal conditions are equally in control of these processes under abnormal conditions.

"Disease" is as natural as health and is as much a manifestation of life as health. It is not something apart from the living organism, not something outside of the functions of life. It is not a something — an *entity* — that is at war with us. "Disease" is not an *attack* upon the body. It is merely one phase of physiological and biological behavior. It is a physiological corrective — abnormal, but not unnatural.

All of the functional and structural changes seen in the organism both in health and "disease" are possible because the body possesses an inherent capacity for complex and continuous adjustment to variable environmental circumstances and internal conditions. These adjustments are variable and not fixed or sterotyped, and are subordinated to the general physiological condition, rather than to external circumstances and emergencies.

Physiology Vs. Voodooism

More than ninety years have passed since Dr. Trall wrote in the introduction to his major work that "the only foundation of a true medical practice is correct physiological principles (for, he says, a "successful practice of the healing art must be based upon the laws of life"); and here is precisely where the whole orthodox medical system of the present day fails —utterly and totally fails. It has no physiological science upon which to practice truly the healing art. In the language of the greatest of modern physiologists, Majendie, 'there is scarcely a sound physiological principle extant'."

Physiology has been much advanced since that statement was made and today we hear much boasting about the progress in this field. Yet, to this day, physiology has not supplied us with a basis for medical practice. It is true that there is often some effort made to correlate some particular medical procedure with physiology, but the physician who makes the attempt is well aware, or should be, that his procedure has no relation to physiology and every intelligent person who views the effort is at once aware of the strained relationship.

In the Aug. 22, 1934 issue of *The Listener*, issued by the British Broadcasting Company, is published under the title "The Frustration of Medicine", a radio address by V. H. Mottram, Professor of Physiology in the University of London, in which he says: "We may confidently assert that in ninety-nine cases out of a hundred he (the medical graduate) sloughs his scientific training when he enters the wards. In fact he is often advised to forget all the physiology which he has learned. Possibly this advice is wise, for it is to be doubted if it is of the slightest use to him."

There seems to me to be but two reasons why a knowledge of physiology can be of no use to the medical practitioner. These are either that (1) the physiology is largely false, or (2) the work he does in practice has no normal relation to physiology. I take the position that the first of these propositions is largely true and that the second is almost wholly so.

Let us look at them in the order given above. Trall said: "When I intimate that there is no physiology in the world, I mean, of course, the medical world. Out of the regular profession this science has been more prospered. Untrammeled by the theories of the schools, individuals, not of the order of medical men, have, as I shall hereafter show, demostrated the true science of life, • • • ."

That statement was published in 1851 and since that time several of the physiological principles announced by Trall and his co-workers have found their way into the regular text-books of physiology. Some of the principles developed by Jennings have only in recent years found their way into biology. Within recent years the so-called rhythm method of birth control has been widely publicized and credit for its discovery given to two men now living. Trall's name is not mentioned in connection with it, but any reader can find the method discussed in Vol. 2 of Trall's work published in 1851.

One of the greatest of living physiologists tells us that teachers and text-book writers of physiology follow a certain pattern laid down by Ludwig's text-book of over eighty years ago.

He says: "one thing, however, is pretty clear — that the information supplied with regard to the central or 'elementary' problems of physiology is often so vague as to be of little apparent practical importance."

In an effort to explain this defect in physiological teaching, he says: "One might at first suppose that whatever general theoretical opinions might be held by a physiological teacher, yet the facts of the science itself must be the same, and that in teaching the facts to the best of his ability, he must be doing all that is possible. But here comes the question, what facts? The facts recorded by physiologists are absolutely infinite in number, and only the more important ones can be taught. Hence in accordance with the general plan just alluded to, only those facts which bear on the 'mechanisms' of the various physiological processes can be taught. If, for instance, we are teaching the physiology of the kidneys, we must teach the main facts bearing on the possible mechanism of secretion of urine. We must thus discuss the possible influence of filtration, diffusion, etc., in the process, leaving out of account all details which are irrelevant to the discussion; and when at the end it turns out that the essential mechanism of secretion is quite unknown there is nothing further to do than pass on to the next subject."

Not only is it true that physiology is taught according to a certain vogue, established over eighty years ago when physiology was just beginning, and all facts ignored that do not fit into the vogue; but it is also true that it is taught as a laboratory science and its relation to life and living are left out. It is an abstract and not a practical science.

There is much in physiology that is pure guesswork. Often we are taught several theo-

ries about a particular physiological phenomenon and left to take our choice. Perhaps
all these theories are wrong. There is much in
physiology that is only tentative. There is much
that is false and there are many errors that
grow out of the limitations of present methods
of investigation. There are also faults that grow
out of the stultifying axiom that only conven-
tions are to be accepted as a basis of principle.

Coming, now, to our second proposition, we
would call special attention to the fact that
the practice of medicine developed ages before physiology was ever thought of. There was
no effort to found it on physiological principles. It was founded on principles that are as
far removed from physiology as the principles of astrology are removed from astronomy.
All of its basic premises, which have been
little modified through the ages, were founded in advance of physiology.

The poisonous drugs, vaccines, serums, etc.,
employed on the basis of these non-physiological principles bear no normal relation to physiology. Their use cannot be justified on physiological grounds. They are anti-vital and anti-
physiological. The same may be said with
equal force for their use of destructive rays.

Their habit of removing organs from the
body and thus depriving it of important physiological structures cannot be supported on
any basis of physiology. It is not to be wondered at that the medical graduates slough their
scientific training when they enter the wards,
for the practices in the wards had their origin
in voodooism, not in science. No wonder they
are advised to forget all they have learned about
physiology, for what they are to do in the wards
has no basis in physiology.

Dr. Mottram, himself, says in this same lecture of the things the medical student is taught in college: "He will not obtain a general oversight of the problems of health and disease as he will meet them in practice. He will obtain a distorted view of the prevalence of venereal diseases. He will learn next to nothing of psychology, of sex, or of diet, three subjects of the utmost importance in private practice. He will go out into practice to find that half his cases suffer for psychological reasons, from faulty sex adjustments and faulty diet, and that a large proportion of the rest of them are due to minor infections of the respiratory tracts."

The Professor concludes that "in no real science would fads and fashions, comparable with those which beset medicine, be possible, or would nostrums, such as the majority of patent medicines and patent foods, hold the field as they do in medicine."

"Medicine," therefore, is not a real science. Medical training fails utterly to equip the student to deal with the most common problems he will meet in practice. Prof. Mottram says the graduate goes out into practice and finds that half of his cases are due to psychological, sexual and dietary maladjustments, but, if our observation is dependable, they never really find this out. They are kept too busy drugging symptoms and cutting out organs to ever study and discover causes. Few of them, apparently, ever do any effective thinking after they leave college. All of them use all the new *cures* turned out by the drug companies. They employ the nostrums, old and new, and keep in step with the passing fads and fashions. A physician recently remarked to me that most physicians learn what to do for their patients from the newspapers.

The Story of Useless Organs

In its early days, its infancy as distinguished from its present pre-adolescence, Biology was cared for by a group of ignorant and semi-ignorant nurse maids who were fond of telling it fairy tales, ghost stories and funny jokes and who answered its many questions about life by telling it the old, familiar story of the stork and how it drops little babies down the chimneys.

One of these nurse maids to biology was a gentleman named Lamark. He worked out a very elaborate and, what proved later to be, a very troublesome, theory about the manner in which species of plants and animals originate. His theory was published in 1809. The big point in his theory of life was the effects of use and disuse. Use develops an organ (he never stopped to explain how an organ can be used before it is developed) and disuse results in its atrophy. He assumed that these effects of use and disuse are hereditary.

Now, there are a lot of organs in the body, the functions of which were then unknown. Most, if not all, of them were small. These were arbitrarily pronounced useless organs. Being both useless and small, what more reasonable than to explain that they had atrophied from disuse. They had been functional in remote ancestors of the race, it was explained, but had fallen into disuse and, as a consequence, had all but disappeared.

The argument ran about this way: "Undeveloped and functionless organs are atrophied organs. But atrophy is the result of disuse. Now disuse presupposes former use. Consequently rudimentary organs were at one time developed and functioning. viz., in the remote ancestors of the race. Since, therefore, these self-same organs are developed and functional in the lower forms of life, it follows that the higher forms, in which these organs are reduced and functionless, are descended from forms similar to those in which said organs are developed and fully functional."

All of these assumptions, utterly at variance with the facts as they are, were taken over from Lamark by Darwin who attached great importance to the existence of "rudimentary organs" in man. Darwin ran up against some hard facts that were opposed to the theory so he invented an ingenious expedient to save his argument. He invented *nascent* organs. These are undeveloped organs which "are of high service to their possessors" and "are capable of further development" and, therefore have a future before them. Rudimentary organs, on the other hand, have had a past but have no future. Unfortunately, "It is however, often (sic) difficult to distinguish between rudimentary and nascent organs, for we can judge only by analogy whether a part is capable of further development, in which case alone it deserves to be called nascent."

Nineteenth Century "science" continued, arbitrarily to pronounce organs useless if their functions were unknown. Darwin, a child of his age, accepted as facts these ignorant pronouncements of "science," and, while acting as nursemaid to the little child, Biology, repeated to the little. fellow these fairy tales of Lamark.

Large numbers of highly serviceable, even indispensable, organs were catalogued as destitute of function, therefore rudimentary, merely because the science of the time had failed to discover their function. They based their arguments on their ignorance and out of this ignorance, they built up a whole series of dogmas that still hamper the progress of biology.

Wallace had warned that "much of what we suppose to be useless is due to our ignorance." Darwin later accepted this same view, saying in the fifth edition of his *Origin of Species,* "I am convinced from the light gained during even the last few years that very many structures which now appear to us useless will hereafter be proved to be useful;" and Wallace, again, referring to "useless" parts gave it his opinion that the assertion of lack of function in the case of any organ or peculiarity which is not a rudiment or a correlation is not, and never can be, the statement of a fact but merely the expression of our ignorance of its purpose or origin.

These men and their echoes and subalterns, however, were so busy putting up walls ahead of foundations and building imposing scientific edifices on the now so well known "we may well believe," or "it may well be supposed," that neither they nor their followers heeded these warnings.

The number of "useless" structures in the human body grew by leaps and bounds until more than two hundred were listed. All of them were referred to "some unknown ancestor" that became extinct long ages ago and neglected to leave any trace of himself in the rocks. Thus it was that these "vestiges," these "rudiments," these "remnants" came to be called "living fossils." It was an evolution by losses, for not one of these "rudiments" was ever regarded as the beginning of a new organ that would, sometime in the future, become a functioning organ. They were always relics of the past and never prophecies of the future.

Among these functionless organs were the tonsils, the vermiform appendix, "that very puzzling organ — the thyroid body," all the other ductless glands, the spleen, etc. The function of the thyroid gland was unknown; hence it had no function. The function of the tonsils was not known; hence, they were without function. The function of the appendix was not known, therefore, it had no function. Ignorance of function was evidence of absence of function.

How explain the presence of functionless organs? That was easy to men who gathered their knowledge from the air and whose crude conceptions of the complexity of physiology makes them seem childish. They were hangovers from organs that once served our "remote ancestors." Those "remote ancestors" needed their functions, whatever these functions may have been; we don't. They have gradually atrophied from disuse.

Older works on evolution would trace for us what was called the "history of the Pineal eye" — a third and unpaired eye, man, in common with many other animals, was supposed to have once possessed. They would actually point out on the lizards, a particular bright scale in the center of the forehead, that represented the former location of the "Pineal eye."

All these discussions of this long-lost "eye" involved a consideration of the "pineal body" connected with the mid-brain of vertebrate animals. This body, which had "long puzzled anatomists" was regarded by "many investigators" as "vestigial." They thought, in other words, that it was the atrophied remains of a structure that "was of some functional value in the ancestors of existing vertebrata." One of the older works says very emphatically: "The truth of this opinion has been demonstrated by the admirable researches of de Graaf and Baldwin Spencer."

That "pineal body," gentle reader, that was an eye in some hypothetical ancestor of vertebrate animals that lived millions of years ago, but which has left no trace of itself and which has no counterpart in any known invertebrate, living or fossil, is the much talked of Pineal gland or *epiphysis*. Instead of it being a functionless remnant of a once useful organ (an eye), this little body is a vitally useful organ. Indeed, its usefulness is out of all proportion to its size.

This median eye, as the "pineal eye" was sometimes called, was lost and we were gravely informed that "it is not unreasonable to suppose that the gradual development and greater utility of the lateral eyes (these are the ones we and other vertebrate animals now use to see with) have led to the suppression of the median eye."

The philosopher Descartes regarded the pineal body as the "seat of the soul," while the evolutionists insisted that "the pineal body in man is clearly vestigial." They warned us, however, that "it is by no means harmless, for occasionally it enlarges and becomes occupied by tumors, sometimes of large size and complex constitution, which cause death from mechanical interference with the brain."

There is a whole group of organs in man which constitute an important regulatory and coordinative system, called the *cryptorhetic system* and made up of ductless or internally secreting glands (*endocrine* glands) which secrete *hormones*, practically all of which were declared to be useless rudiments.

The pineal gland (*epiphysis*) the pituitary gland (*hypophysis*), the thyroid gland, the parathyroid glands, the thymus gland, the adrenal glands (supra-renal capsules), etc., were all said to be functionless.

The paramount importance of these glands is now well known. For instance, in man and other animals, death follows immediately upon the removal of the adrenal glands. Likewise, complete removal of the thyroid produces death. The secretions of each and all of these glands are vitally important to life and development.

We were told that man, "in common with the four anthropomorphous apes" has a small thin tube, varying in length from two to eight inches, attached to the lower end of the coecum, called the vermiform appendix. Man, apes, gibbons and the little wombat are the only mammals possessed of an appendix. Now this appendix has no function. This assertion is based on the well established principle: *if no function is known, none exists.* We were told that the appendix in the newly-born child is often absolutely (and not merely relatively) as long as in the full-grown man and, then, we were gravely assured that "this precocity is always an indication that the part was of great importance to the ancestors of the human species."

I leave it to the reader to guess how they found out that "this precocity" has this significance. I have never been able to discover how they discovered the truth of this dogma. Perhaps they discovered it in the same realm in which they discovered that the appendix has no function — in the realm of ignorance. "It may well be supposed" that the appendix, which "we may confidently believe" now has no function, was once of great use to some pre-ape ancestor of man. And "it is not unreasonable to suppose" that precocity indicates something or other.

The appendix of the anthropormophous (man-like) apes has no function — this for the same reason that man's appendix has no function — i.e., its function is unknown.

The other mammals (except some carnivores: In the carnivores, such as lions and tigers, there is no coecum and the appendix is said to be "more vestigial than in man.") do not possess an appendix. They possess, instead, a very large coecum and "in some of these terminal segments of the coecum, although not represented as a thin, narrow tube, nevertheless resembles the vermiform appendix in that it possesses a very large proportion of the peculiar kind of tissue known as adenoid or lymphatic." They would have found much more of this adenoid tissue if they had given a little attention to the omentum.

Thus it was that they "discovered" that the vermiform appendix is the vestigial remains of a once large and functioning coecum. The coecum and the appendix both have a large amount of lymph-adenoid tissue. Now the oracle speaks. In deep tones that indicate authority, it says: "In man the vermiform appendix is a typical example of a functionless part."

In his *Descent of Man*, Darwin says: "With respect to the alimentary canal, I have met with an account of only a single rudiment, namely, the vermiform appendix of the coecum. ••• Not only is it useless, but it is sometimes the cause of death, of which fact I have lately heard two instances. This is due to small hard bodies, such as seeds, entering the passage and causing inflammation."

Every assumption in the above quotation is false. The appendix is a functioning organ; it never causes death; and, to quote the famous surgeon, Dr. John B. Deaver, "The old idea that foreign bodies, such as grape seeds, are the cause of the disease (appendicitis) has been disproved."

All "vestigal" structures were considered to be potential sources of danger. Thus, the "functionless" appendix, "like an idle person in a community, is not infrequently a source of danger and suffering, and is responsible for a number of deaths annually."

This language reveals how much of its sustenance biology drew from the medical teat to which it fixed itself, like a parasite, and from which it has not yet detached itself. Perhaps this parasitism accounts for the failure of its brain to develop.

The appendix was (or is) a source of danger and suffering and causes many deaths annually. Does this not put the cause of disease in the wrong place? Does this not make the organ most involved the cause of the trouble? Is this not the medical idea, even to this day? So long as Biology clings to the medical teat and draws its "intellectual" pap from this source, it will never become a true science of life.

The appendix was held to be a threefold source of danger:

(1) Its opening into the coecum may become closed and the tube distended into a cyst in consequence of fluid accumulating within it. "Such a cyst may rupture, and lead to minor troubles, as local inflammation or abscess, or induce death by peritonitis." This "danger" seems to be more theoretical than real.

(2) "A much commoner danger is the entrance into it of fruit stones and similar indigestible substances taken with the food; these act as irritants, and in the long run destroy life." Grape seed, tomato seed, small shot, even cherry seed, and other such substances were supposed to get into and lodge in the appendix. In lions and tigers, with still "more vestigal" appendices, they told stories of finding nails, pieces of wood, bones and stones in the appendix. This "cause" for appendicitis is no longer accepted.

(3) "Adenoid or lymphatic tissue," it was explained, "is very prone to ulcerate, and under certain conditions the adenoid tissue lining the appendix may inflame and lead to fatal perforation." This danger was supposed to be much less common than trouble arising from cherry stones, grape pits, tomato seed, small shot, etc., finding lodgement in the lumen of the appendix.

The tonsils also, were said to be "often the seat of disease which is not merely troublesome to the individual, but is at times fraught with great danger to life." All of this emphasis on the fact that supposedly functionless or "vestigal" organs are "often the seat of disease" that is "not merely troublesome," but also, "at times fraught with great danger to life," is a puzzle. There is no part of the body that is not "often the seat" of "troublesome" and "dangerous" disease. Functional or "functionless" — all parts become sick.

The above quotation about the tonsils was said about the faucial tonsils. Of these they said: "Structurally they are composed of adenoid tissue, covered with mucous membrane, beset with a number of shallow crypts which secrete thick, tenacious mucus." There is nothing in their structure to indicate that they are functionless. So, they take a look at their locations. "The niche in which each (faucial) tonsil is lodged is termed the tonsillar recess, and indicates the exact spot where the second branchial cleft in the embryo communicated with the pharynx."

Now this branchial cleft is one of those so-called gill-slits seen at a certain stage of our embryonic development that was once thought to be sure proof that we are descended from fish. One of these "gill-slits" when its development is completed, becomes the tympano-eustachian passage, the small tubercules surmounting it becoming the external ear.

It seems that the location of the faucial tonsils at the "exact spot where the second bronchial cleft in the embryo communicated with the pharynx," indicates that the tonsils are useless structures. The origin and location of the ears should indicate that they, too, are functionless. Perhaps they would, were the function of the ear unknown. The functions of the tonsils were unknown so it was assumed they had no function. There were other proofs of this. "How far the tonsils subserve any useful purpose is very doubtful: Certainly they are often removed, and persons usually experience relief rather than suffer inconvenience from the loss."

Discussing "gutteral or eustachian pouches" seen on horses, we are told that they are probably "dilatations of the pharyngeal ends of the second branchial clefts. These are the clefts from which the tonsils of man arise. It is also of some importance to remember that in the early human embryo the tonsil is represented as a sac with a slit-like opening wherewith it communicates with the pharynx." Then comes the final proof of the inutility of the tonsils: "like the tonsils of man, they are sources of inconvenience, trouble, and occasionally disaster. Like the tonsils, also, no known function is served by these pouches." Horses have no faucial tonsils.

In passing, it may be well to list the development from these five pairs of alleged gill-slits seen at a certain stage of the development of the human embryo. These are:

  1. The Eustachian tubes; one from the throat to each ear.

  2. The palatine, or faucial tonsils.

  3. The thymus gland.

  4. The parathyroid glands.

  5. The post-branchial bodies.

The functionless character of these structures is no longer affirmed on the basis of ignorance of function or that of their "origin."

Man has other tonsils besides the faucial tonsils. One of these, "the pharyngeal tonsil of Luschka, in honor of its discoverer," is "structurally, identical with the tonsils." "As far as is at present known, this organ has no function, but is often a source of trouble and inconvenience, mainly in children, inasmuch as it is especially prone to enlarge and obstruct the eustachian tube, producing deafness. It also interferes, when large, with the free passage of air through the nostrils, to such a degree as to require surgical interference."

This pharyngeal tonsil is commonly called "adenoids." Why call it adenoids? Because it is composed of adenoid tissue. The throat is full of adenoid tissue. Indeed, this tissue, in the form of lymph nodes and lymph nodules (commonly referred to as lymph glands), Pyer's patches, etc., is distributed throughout the body. It is a very useful tissue, forming part of the body's first line of defense against poisons and "infections." Instead of being functionless, its function is very essential to life and health and is as continuous as the circulation of the blood.

In his *History of the Human Body*, H. H. Wilder points out that in the tonsils, the lymphatic nodules of the intestines, the thymus gland and other aggregations of adenoid tissues in the body, the the lymphocytes (lymph cells or white blood corpuscles) have their origin. The *appendix vermiformis*, besides secreting a lubricating fluid for the colon, probably shares with all other lymph-adenoid tissue throughout the body, the work of destroying toxins and that of producing *lymphocytes*.

There are other "useless" organs which I have not mentioned, such as the supposed rudimentary tail of man (the coccyx), the "rudimentary" nictitating membrane of the eye, etc. Both the above named structures have definite functions. The advance of physiology has rapidly depleted the list of useless organs until,today, there remain but a few and in these their days of "uselessness" are numbered. As rudiments they will soon be forgotten. Perhaps if a reactionary "science" had not discouraged investigation into their functions, by its dogmatic assertion that they were rudiments and had no function, their functions would have been dicovered before now.

The Fun of Being Sick

I once read of a woman, who, upon being asked by her physician on one of his frequent visits, how she was feeling, replied: "I am enjoying my sickness, thank you." Please don't think of that as a mere joke; it is all too tragically true. We are a world of sick men and women who "enjoy our sickness."

Psychologists talk very learnedly about the "will to live" and kill themselves as early as do the common herd. If there is a "will to live" the evidence for it must be very small. The sick die — many of them take a longer time than others to finish the process, but, dying, they all ultimately die.

Only the well can live. Barring violence, they can live as long as they remain well. But who wants to be well? Who wants to live if he must give up his sickness in order to do so? A "will to live" would involve, or be correlated with, a "will to be well" and this would involve a "will to live well."

We don't live well and don't want to do so. We want to "enjoy life," and this means being sick all of our short lives. By "enjoying life," we don't mean life, we mean *indulgencies*. By "enjoyment" we mean experiencing all forms of unnatural and abnormal thrills, sensations and irritations.

The following from a letter from one of our students and subscribers tells a story that may be duplicated in every office, shop, store, and most modern homes in America. The lady who writes the letter is an artist, a portrait painter, who is now doing art work of some different kind for the war effort. She was a student in my classes given in New York on several of my visits to that city. She is one of the few who made use of what she learned and did not permit herself to be carried away by the next Hindu spellbinder or the next seller of patent foods who came to town. Perhaps this was due to the fact that she had already tried them all and found them to be false teachers. But to her letter:

"I always have felt the most fortunate of humans to have learned from you the truths on health I had sought to know for so many years before I studied with you. I had so much material (and a general knowledge of the subject that was helpful to be sure) but nevertheless so confusing that I am eternally grateful to you for unraveling the maze of contradictions handed me. You have simplified what I sought to know with such amazing clarity that I have always wondered since, why everyone that ever listened to you or read your books could not easily be convinced they were being given the only genuine education in simple healthful living that they would ever need. If·they went no where else to study but merely went along with your little magazine, *Hygienic Review*, from month to month, they would be serving themselves and all those about them·with the best knowledge on the subject available handed them on a silver platter — the real value of its·contents being priceless.

"I paid all kinds of money, years ago for health courses but I was never satisfied as having sufficient foundation so I could use it to live by and continue with complete attention to my work which, as you know is that of an artist. But after having studied with you about 10 or more years ago I was convinced my search was over and being well or otherwise was in my own hands and so long as I obey the simple laws of health that you taught me all's well and when I digress, the results are all too obvious. But there's no mystery about it so that when I again have the conditions for health why there I am back in shape again. I am convinced that if I had adhered to medical standards of treatment I'd have been a dead pigeon long ago.

"I have had some very serious accidents. Ten years ago they said I'd never walk again. I disproved that after a few weeks though I had to walk slowly for a year. Only last year I fell down a flight of stairs and hurt my spine pretty badly — people called a doctor — he said I'd be laid up for about 6 months at least — I was at work in a week and though it took 6 months to heal completely I was useful in all that time because I lived simply and knew my limitations. From that accident of 10 years ago to this one I had never been away from work for illness.

"Where I work now I am actually the only one who has not been out for illness except after the accident — for a week. We have between 20 and 30 people in our small division of the camp and there are just about that many different ailments. One gets thyroid, another hayfever injections, a third a TB case — collapsed lungs — sinus, kidney trouble, high blood pressure — well, all the rest of ailments that are usually current. One insists on the windows being closed, another insists on them being open, one is forever sneezing, another forever wheezing — there's continuous fear of getting too close to one another for fear of passing on the cold the other has — one coughs so badly each morning that we fear it will be her last and that is not the TB case, either.

"Aspirin is the order of the day. The conversation goes something like this: 'Gee, I feel sick. I've taken 4 aspirins and it hasn't helped me at all.' 'Here, I have some drops, put them into your nose; — they'll help.' 'Take these cough drops, they're the best in the market." And the girl who has the sinus trouble and is always going to the doctor to have them drained, swears by her doctor because she is so much relieved after each drainage — and when I mention about her food habits being bad and her chain smoking she says its ridiculous that they have any bearing on her trouble or her doctor would have told her so. The other girl who has anemia and a catarrhal condition so bad that the odor of decay is pronounced, brings her lunch of white bread, hard boiled egg, cake and whatnots every day and when I mention foods, why, her answer is there may be something in it, so when she has a piece of apple or orange that someone shares she says 'see this is for you' — to appease me.

"I could go on telling you how the Coca-Cola machines are forever being emptied — every few minutes someone says 'cokes?' and nickels are handed in and someone goes out to get them — where they put it all is beyond me. And the candy machines are emptied just as often. I have seen a worm in the peanut candy that was a bright green and an inch long — jump out as the bar was broken. A number of people make lunch of a meat sandwich and ice cream nearly every day. One girl has appendicitis 'attacks' so frequently no one pays attention any more and the lady who had the tumor removed and insists that it saved her life, is forever urging this other girl to have that appendix taken out — it's useless, she claims. For some reason the fellow with the hernia gets all the heavy lifting jobs to do though everyone knows he has a hernia and is out of the Army for that reason, plus his punctured ear drum which he says he got from a slip in an examination by some nurse or medic. One fellow has a protuberance growing out of the side of his jaw and the doctor says he has glandular trouble. Another fellow's skin is peeling off his fingers in a peculiar manner and his concession to a change in living habits is one item — just having no sugar in his daily coffee (several times a day). I don't believe there's one there that doesn't have at least 3 cups a day while at work. They go out morning, noon and afternoon for a cup.

"I know they think me queer but they respect me it seems for the work I do and for the fact that there must be something to what I say; — for I'm not sick like the rest. But they insist I do it *at the expense of not enjoying life* since having a 'thick, juicy steak' means enjoying life to them. And, mind you, these are not unschooled people; they are college graduates, engineers and nearly everyone is outstanding in the work he or she does and people so cultivated in any number of fields that one is enriched in many ways by being with them. They are the kindliest folk one could meet. They know everything but the most important thing to know — how to keep well."

These people are all convinced that this woman remains well 'at the expense of not enjoying life." On the other hand, they are enjoying their sickness. Their habits are an integral part of their sickness just as her habits are an integral part of her health. We cannot divorce life from living.

But these poor highly educated ignoramuses don't really enjoy their coffee, Coca-Cola, candy, cigarettes, etc. They take these things for the same reason they employ aspirin, cough drops, insulin, thyroid extracts and sinus drainages — they can't bear their unpleasant sensations when they are not under the influence of such drugs. They use tobacco, coffee, coca-cola, candy, etc., to smother their symptoms — their discomforts —and to cover up their miseries. They prefer re-narcotization to their suffering when not narcotized.

Tobacco doesn't give them pleasure; it only temporarily smothers their discomforts. Coffee doesn't give them enjoyment; it temporarily "relives" their headaches and stimulates (irritates) them so that they don't feel tired. Coca Cola, containing the same drug (caffeine) as coffee, has the same effect.

Note the number of bottles of Coca-Cola and the number of cups of coffee they each have daily and you will get an idea of how firmly they are in the grasp of the caffeine habit — caffeine addiction. They are drug addicts and they think they are enjoying life. They are sick and they think they are enjoying life. They are neurotics and they think they are enjoying their neuroses.

They run to physicians who dose them and cut them and inoculate them to "cure" them or "relieve" them of the effects of their "enjoyment" and they imagine they are educated. They are products of an education that doesn't educate.

A French philosopher is reported to have said that "the art of living is the art of making a damned fool of oneself." He is said to have advised: "never let another make an ass of you: do it yourself." I think he must have had in mind the people who "enjoy life" as the above educated and cultured ignoramuses "enjoy" it. They would seem to be doing a good job of following his advice.

Nature's decree, inexorably even if not always swiftly executed, is this: THE STUPID SHALL PERISH.

How to Get Well

Dr. Tilden has well said that "palliating suffering under the guise of curing leads an appetite-and-passion-crazed civilization to its doom."

Living generations, "old" and young have dedicated their lives to indulgence and the commercial crowd, intent only upon gaining ever increasing profits, finds it very profitable to stimulate and aid them in sticking to their consecration. The mad chase after the pleasures and thrills of appetite and passion cannot fail to produce a rich harvest of disease and premature death. Who cares?

Do you know of a college faculty the members of which will not die prematurely because they do not know enough to live out a reasonable life expectancy? Are they not all satisfied with an expectancy based on lying statistics? Have they not all accepted and are they not content with a low standard of health based on low conditions?

If our educators, our wise men, do not know how to live, who does? Do the doctors of the various schools? Are they not all sick? Do they not die prematurely? Are they not addicted to all the conventional or popular indulgencies and bad habits? Are their families healthy? Do you know of one who sells cures that cure? Do you know of one teaching reform that reforms?

Health is the supreme virtue and it cannot be experienced by one addicted to disease-producing habits. Reform means giving up habits that build disease and produce premature death. It means cultivating habits that build health and prolong life. If sickness follows reform, it shows that the reform is not real. Either the reformed is a weakling or a hypocrite — he is a cheat, a liar, a pretender, a dissembler, an imposter—else his teacher and advisor is a fake and a humbug.

"The only cure-all is to correct disease-producing habits." says Tilden. "Because disease is built by enervating habits — when habits are given up, health follows." Because disease is built by enervating habits, health cannot follow so long as enervating habits are practiced.

"Curing" disease does not produce health. Palliating symptoms does not restore health. Cutting out affected organs does not restore health. None of the methods and systems of prevention, cure and palliation do more than palliate effects; they do not remove, or even regard, cause. They are outside of life, not parts of life, but artificial and enforced superadditions to life that produce their own evils.

Cures are not only failures, they are unnecessary evils. Disease is built by enervating habits — when enervating habits are discontinued the sick get well. If habits have been persisted in so long and disease has been allowed to last until organic change has occurred, a competent *Hygienist* will be needed to guide the sick person back to health. The doctor or physician who neglects to help his patient break off the habits that produced the organic change will fail. His palliative treatments will add to the pathology. Nature will cure when the patient and treater get rid of disease-provoking habits and treatments.

What the sick need is teachers not treaters, health schools not hospitals, instruction not treatment, education in right living not training the sick habit. Both they and their advisors must get rid of the *curing* idea and the practices built up thereon.

Simple diseases continue and develop into formidable pathological conditions under continuous treatment, because doctors of all schools ignore enervating habits. They try to cure disease in spite of a mode of living that builds disease daily. They will not learn the truth, either because they are too stupid or because commercialism and racketeering have become the dominating power over their minds and lives.

Have we a reader so stupid that he is unable to understand that to remove the cause is the only way to get rid of an effect? If man builds his disease by practicing enervating habits, how can he get well if he does not stop the enervating habits? If he returns to his habits, the disease is soon rebuilt.

To medicate and palliate — to relieve discomfort — to cut out organs and parts of organs, to "cure" disease instead of removing cause, that is, instead of correcting life, is foolish. It is like applying an ointment to the foot in which a tack is sticking instead of removing the tack.

Removing corns will not remove the cause of corns. Removal of inflamed tonsils does not remove the cause of the inflammation. Removing a tumor or a cancerous growth does not remove the cause of tumor or cancer. To remove or palliate any symptom does not remove cause. Until cause is removed no recovery is possible. When cause is removed nature restores health, nature removes the effect.

Doing Something

Thomas L. Nichols, M.D., made a place for himself among the pioneers in the *Hygienic movement*. He was a medical student at Dartmouth when Sylvester Graham went to Boston to lecture in the 1830's. That was more than a hundred years ago. Nichols attended Graham's lectures and became convinced that medicine was all wrong. He gave up his medical studies and became editor of the New York *Evening Herald*.

In New York in the 1840's he met Mary Gove, a remarkable woman who had been the first woman to prepare herself to lecture on *Hygiene*, or, as it was commonly known at that time, Grahamism. Mrs. Gove was attracted by the *Water Cure* and went to New York to acquaint herself with its principles. After sometime spent in the Water Cure establishment of Dr. Joel Shew, she opened a *Water Cure* of her own in New York, at that time but a small town.

In those days no woman was permitted to attend Medical College and there were no other schools of "healing" to attend. Nichols decided that since Mrs. Gove could not get a license to practice, he would complete his studies of medicine, secure a license and share it with her, thus protecting her in her work. Their marriage came in due course as did his degree in medicine and his license.

Nichols studied medicine in the University of New York under the famous Dr. Valentine Mott. He would often laugh to himself over the thought of the revolutionary purposes to which he was going to put the reactionary knowledge they dispensed at this place. Nichols graduated near the head of his class.

In the spring of 1850 Dr. Thomas and Mary Gove Nichols moved to 87 W. 22nd St., with their establishment where they did a flourishing work for a number of years, before they went to England where they spent the remainder of their days. When asked what was the difference between their "Water Cure" and that of Dr. Shew, Mary Gove Nichols would reply: "To us, Water Cure is Love Cure."

This remarkable couple were the first psychoanalysts. It is doubtful that they ever employed the term, using instead the term, *esoteric anthropology*, but they employed its technique and formulated a sound theory as a basis for their psychoanalytic work. Two of our contemporary historians say that the term employed by the Nicholses is "a more accurate descriptive title than the later and more generally used term psychoanalysis. Furthermore, they knew that their methods came straight from Mesmer, a knowledge lacking in the Freudians of today."

In a future article I shall discuss Dr. Nichols' formulation of his, or rather, the *Hygienic*, theory of the cause of disease. At this time I desire to confine myself largely to what he says about the *do something* principle of the schools of medicine. He says:

"The first thing we must learn—the first principle of medicine, and the one most often disregarded, is to do no mischief. It is not true that *we must do something*. Unless we know what to do, it is always safer and better *to do nothing*. If we are not sure that we can aid nature, we must not run the risk of hindering her with our interference. All experience shows that, in a great majority of cases, she effects a cure without assistance, and even in spite of mischievous efforts." (The italics are his.)

"To do nothing," he says, "is better than to do mischief." He quotes the following statement made by Napoleon to the Italian physician, Autonomarchi; "Believe me, we had better leave off all these remedies. Life is a fortress which neither you nor I know anything about. Why throw obstacles in the way of its defense? Its own means are superior to all the apparatus of your laboratories. Covisart candidly agreed with me that all your filthy mixtures are good for nothing. Medicine is a collection of uncertain prescriptions, the results of which, taken collectively, are more fatal than useful to mankind. Water, air, and cleanliness are the chief articles in my pharmacopoeia."

"If medicine were only as wise as surgery!" exclaims Dr. Nichols. "When a man has a broken bone, the surgeon is content to put it in place, prescribe rest, and a moderate diet, and leave nature to mend it. But when it is the liver or lungs that are disordered, the doctor bleeds and blisters, and doses, gives alterative, cathartic, opiate, and does more mischief in a week than nature can remedy in a year."

Although, as he so truly said, "all experience shows that in a great majority of cases, she (nature) effects a cure without assistance, and even in spite of mischievous efforts," what is (what was) the practice of the sick, their families, nurses and physicians? Let Dr. Nichols tell us. He says:

"But the moment anyone is taken ill — that is, the moment nature begins the operation of expelling some matter of disease — everybody wants to do something to the patient. Every old woman rushes in with her infallible nostrum, and nature, who has honestly set to work to cure a disease, finds herself hindered on every side. When the stomach is incapable of digestion, it must be deluged with gruels, rice water, and barley water, as if the moment one was sick, he was in imminent danger of starvation. Then comes the doctor, and if one of the common sort, the attack begins in earnest. A few years ago out came the lancet, and followed its rude gash a quart of blood. Poor nature, feeling the work she had to do, and needing all her strength, gasped at this murderous sacrifice; but the next attack was to cover fifty square inches of skin with a torturing blister, and at the same time to pour down the throat doses of the most virulent poisons of the *materia medica*. This went on, and when nature finally sunk under the disease, and the added enthusiasm of a vile torturing medication, everybody consoled himself with the idea that 'everything was done that could be done'; it should be added, 'to kill the patient'."

The practice of so-called medicine has undergone some change, due largely to pressure from the outside, since Dr. Nichols wrote, but it can hardly be said to have improved much. It no longer bleeds its victims to death. Instead of blood-letting being the universal cure-all, blood transfusions are rapidly becoming the *panacea*. Powerful poisons are still in use, while surgery has grown into a greater menace to the sick than has medicine.

"I have no patience with the folly of patients," says Dr. Nichols, "or the ignorance, to call it no worse, of physicians. But when I see how the latter are educated, and the former deceived, I cannot wonder at the result. I have seen hundreds of medical students; I have attended the lectures of two medical colleges. 'I speak what I know, and I testify what I have seen.' What Napoleon said is true of the highest and most enlightened. What, then, must be the truth respecting the great mass of medical practitioners?"

The frantic, almost hysterical *doing something* that goes on so industriously at the bedside of the sick is the cause of thousands of deaths yearly. Have you not seen the wringing of hands and heard the hysterical cry: "Why doesn't somebody do something?" Anything, just so something is being done. The physicians of the world meet this demand in thousands of destructive ways.

"To do nothing is better than to do mischief," says Nichols, "but it is not so well as to do something that should be done. When a man has fallen into a ditch, we had better do nothing than jump upon him and bury him deeper; but it is much better to carefully pull him out, cleanse him of the mud, put him in the right path, and send him on his way rejoicing."

"We can do all that is practicable to remove the cause of disease," he explains. But removing cause is not enough. Physicians and treaters insist on *doing* something — something *curative*. The patient and members of his family all insist that *something should be done. Do something!* This is the universal cry. And they are never satisfied until they have been *done* to death.

Why Drugs?

Some few years since an article was published in this country from the pen of Sir William Arbuthnot Lane, who is considered one of the greatest living British physicians and surgeons, under the title "Why Drugs Are Necessary."

Although, in this article Sir William failed to explain why drugs are necessary, if they are, he did tell us in a very emphatic manner that we are not to think that all drug treatment is scientifically futile and that we must not think that drugs have no place in the curative resources of the "scientific" physician. He says that the "pharmacopeia has been drastically expurgated and only those drugs whose precise effect upon the body is known are now included."

This statement is perfectly meaningless. The pharmacopea still carries a great amount of trash. Be this as it may, the drugs that are now must popular with physicians are those that are most powerful in their effects. It is still true that "our strongest poisons are our best remedies."

The fact that the "precise effect" of a drug is known does not justify its use in treating the sick. For, whatever else it may do, it can in no wise aid in correcting or removing the cause of disease, nor can it contribute in any way to the healthful functions of the organism.

Drugs all produce several effects and not just a precise effect. Medical men regard only the primary and temporary drug effects in writing their prescriptions and take no account of the secondary and lasting effects.

Sir William says: "Pharmacological science has also given us preparations which are pure and standardized."

Pure what? Pure poisons! Elements and compounds that are foreign to the body and that should never be introduced therein!

Standardized preparations! Perhaps so! But who or what supplies the standardized patients? How can we have a standardized treatment without a standardized patient?

He further says: "Generally speaking, and contrary to popular opinion, drugs are not given to act upon diseased tissues but on healthy ones."

This fact, if it is a fact, is certainly no reason for employing drugs. Contrary, however, to medical opinions, drugs do not act on diseased or healthy tissues in anything like the manner they think they do. They have no selective action that enables them to pass up the diseased tissue and act only upon the healthy tissue. Indeed, as between lifeless and living matter, the former is passive, the latter is active. The relation between the living tissues of the body and lifeless or inorganic drug is one of eternal antagonism.

It is the living system that does the acting — it is the lifeless drug that is acted upon. All this talk of medical men about the physiological action of drugs is baseless moonshine. They might as well write their books about the "living principles of death" or the "eternal laws of non-existence." Dr. Trall well said "Poisons are pathological — disease producing. Physiological poison and pathological health — healthy poison and sickly health — are equally rational and irrational expressions."

If it is the drug that acts, prove it by securing bowel action in a dead man by administering a strong purgative; give a powerful emetic to the dead and produce vomiting; produce a blister on the body of a fresh corpse by applying a blistering plaster. Why are these "actions" of drugs less in those who are feeble and greater in the strong and vigorous? Why does their "action" grow less as vital resistance is lowered?

Their "action" is precisely in proportion to the vigor, integrity and resisting power of the living and acting organism. And this is so because these so-called therapeutic actions of drugs are the actions of the body in resisting and expelling the drugs. It is their hostility to life that causes drugs to appear to act. Their apparent action is in proportion to their hostility to the body's welfare.

Looking more closely at the supposed actions of "remedies", let us emphasize that they never produce any functional result whatever. It is not the cathartic that purges, or the emetic that vomits, or the diaphoretic that sweats, or the diuretic that urinates; but these things are eliminated through these channels and by these means.

This is no mere play on words; but a scientific principle of the greatest importance. Many mistakes come from attributing to material agents, functional actions that belong to the living body only. These may excite, but they cannot produce functional activities.

It makes all the difference in the world whether the drug or supposed remedy produces function or is expelled by function. To ignore this distinction is equivalent to ignoring the powers of life; and the next step would be the attempted substitution of cathartics for the colon, diurectics for the kidneys, electricity for life.

Sir William continues, saying "Rest is the sheet anchor of all forms of treatment, for it places a diseased tissue in the best possible position for the restorative processes of nature to operate."

Rest! How little does he know of rest! How can the drugged organism rest? In the very nature of things it must resist the drug and this resistance is not rest. Rest is not a form of treatment and does not belong to any form of treatment. He adds:

"The physician, then, is always aiming at restoring an unhealthy or damaged organ and not infrequently he is able to do this through the medium of a drug."

I have never met a physician of the type he describes and am inclined to think that the physician that Sir William has in mind exists only in his imagination. All the physicians I come in contact with are busy treating symptoms. They are certainly not busy removing or correcting the causes of impaired functions and organs, a thing that no drug can do, and, therefore, no physician can restore health "through the medium of a drug."

Dr. Lane offers, as a prize example of how the physician may employ drugs to restore health, the following: "For example, digitalis is given in disease of the heart valve, not with the intention of repairing the injured valve, but to act upon the healthy heart muscle so obviating the disturbance of the blood circulation occasioned by the deformed valves."

I am sure that Sir William is well aware that digitalis does not restore the heart to normal, but rather makes its condition worse. Nor can its use be continued indefinitely.

It is well known that no drug can be given permanently, but that there comes a point when the use of calomel, antimony, strychnine, quinine. digitalis, etc., must cease, whether or not the purpose for which the doctor administered it has been accomplished. The more delicate the constitution, the weaker the organism, the greater the reduction of strength from the cause of disease, the sooner is this point reached.

When tested at the bedside, drugs become least apparently useful at the point where they should be most needed. For, as the condition of the patient becomes most grave and his body seems to be yielding to the causes of the disease already present (and lacks the power to produce a new form of disease in opposing the drugs of the physician), drugs lose their supposed power to act. At precisely the point where the physician's art would seem to be most urgently needed, the physician is forced to withhold his "curative" or "restful" drugs and leave the case in the hands of nature.

In such cases, if the patient is to recover at all, it is necessary that drugging be abandoned. The frequency with which recovery follows upon the cessation of drugging, in such cases, indicates very strongly that it was the drugs that were killing the patient.

Digitalis is used in many conditions to occasion certain alterations in heart action. In all cases its use is to change the vital manifestations that are labeled disease. In one form or another the idea has prevailed throughout the history of medicine that the vital phenomena of so-called disease constitutes the danger. This one mistake has been the fundamental error that has vitiated medical theory and practice from the beginning. It has lead to the effort to secure quiescence in function without regard to the condition upon which the disturbance depends and without consideration for the object aimed at by the active operation of the vital powers.

The dynamic or vital manifestations are not the danger, but efforts of the body to remove the sources of danger. Increased heart action and increased temperature are both vital phenomena and are in no proper sense any real portion of the danger to the organism, though they are evidences of the existence of danger. These dangerous conditions are certainly to be corrected, but the functional modifications collectively called disease, sequent to these are not, on that account, to be suppressed, subdued, silenced or extinguished by the physician and his "remedies."

The forcible reduction of heart action certainly does not remove the necessity for accelerated circulation. The forcible reduction of temperature does not remove the necessity for the fever. So long as such physiological actions as irritation, fever, inflammation, vomiting, diarrhea, coughing, etc., are regarded as the source of danger, just so long will physicians be justified in sending in their bills as did the old Irish physician who rendered his bill to the bereaved huband of one of his women patients, thus: "For curing your wife until she died, $50.00."

The error that "abnormal" vital actions are evil and dangerous has deprived all who accept it of the power to learn anything certain about the value of their methods of treatment. Nothing can be more ruinous to our logic, nor more damaging in our practice, than to confound a consequence with a cause. To make this mistake in "medical science" is to view the vital actions of so-called disease as the source of danger; is to class life's efforts to restore health as being the very things that endanger life.

The so-called symptoms of disease are manifestations of an inherent principle of the organism to restore healthy function and to resist offending agents and influences. They are salutary efforts of nature to repair an injury or to re-establish health. The cause of fever, inflammation, irritation, like that of all other physiological actions and processes, is always one and the same — namely, the *vital force*. It is because all agents that affect the system for evil, if they do not instantly paralize it, excite it to acts of a physiological character — conservative, defensive, or reparative — which acts are the processes of cure in every case, that we live at all.

To subdue, suppress or "regulate" these vital expressions is to thwart nature's efforts at eliminating the causes of damaged structure and restoring health. Such measures can never restore health, although the body is often able to restore health in spite of them.

Dr. Lane then mentions a class of drugs which "act" on a different principle and "are potent enemies against microbic" disease. Quinine for malaria is included in this list. "In this case," he says, "the quinine acts as a poison to the germ of malaria, killing it."

There is no reason to doubt that quinine is deadly to the supposed malarial parasite, but it is also poisonous to the body of the patient. It does not exercise any selective power and confine its action to the parasites. Neither does its use either prevent or cure malaria.

"Arsenic, bismuth and mercury," he says, "are used to kill the parasites of syphilis." They are so used; this is not denied. We only deny that they kill the supposed parasites before they kill the patient.

Lastly, Sir William reminds us that there is a form of drug treatment known as endocrine therapy, that iron is given in anemia and "vitamin concentrates" are given in deficiency diseases. But he neglected to add that the glandular substances do not correct causes, while they produce troubles of their own; he omitted to mention that giving iron in anemia produces several troubles and does not improve the condition of the blood or remove the cause of the anemia; he failed to say that "vitamin concentrates" are delusions, while natural foods carry all the vitamins needed.

His entire defense of drugs is unworthy of a school child and serves only to remind us that he was brought up in the drug school and will never be able to eradicate its fallacies from his mind. He was baptized in falsity and miseducated throughout the whole of his life, so that the errors I am here combatting have become ingrained and seem to have become parts of him. For a time it looked as though Sir William was regaining sanity and would throw the whole drug system away; but, unfortunately, his recovery was never quite complete.

Toleration

Barring violence, perhaps the only cause of death is tolerated poisoning. The slow, gradual, insidious undermining of the organism — the wasting of its nervous energy and the impairing of its functional and structural integrity — by poisons that are harbored and "tolerated" kills sooner or later. Yet, *toleration* is one of the most misunderstood phenomena in all nature. Very few men and women grasp its true character.

Tolerance for poisoning is established by breaking down resistance to its influence. The body pays for this toleration (miscalled immunity) by general enervation and lowered resistance to every other influence.

It has been objected that the breaking down of resistance should not produce toleration, that it should weaken the organism and render it more susceptible to the influence of poison. This objection arises out of not understanding the phenomena of resistance.

We have seen tolerance defined as the "ability to endure the continued use of a drug." We have also seen it defined as the ability to resist a drug. There is something wrong somewhere. It is one thing to resist; it is another to endure.

That the vital system resists drug poisons is not doubted. The means of resistance are not well understood. When emesis (vomiting) follows a dose of ipecac and diarrhea follows a dose of calomel, these processes are recognized as evidences of intolerance; but they are not understood to be means of resistance. Resistance is supposed to be some occult power that comes into play after the physiological evidences of intolerance have ceased. This is the reason we are told that tolerance means being inured to poison by habit so that it may be taken without harm.

So long as the body actively resists and speedily expels the poison, it is supposed to produce harm, after active resistance has ceased and rapid expulsion no longer occurs, it is supposed to be harmless.

It should be obvious to even a child that its speedy expulsion prevents harm while its toleration permits it to do much harm. If calomel is expelled by diarrhea, it does not get into the blood and cannot damage the blood, nerves, bones, teeth, etc. If it is not expelled by diarrhea, it does get into the blood and does damage all of these structures.

It is a sad day for the body when it learns to tolerate poisons. If intolerance persists it will force cessation of the use of poison. If tolerance for tobacco were never established, there would be no tobacco users. The same may be said of alcohol, opium, arsenic, and other poisons.

Note that the symptoms of poisoning — pain, nausea, vomiting, griping, diarrhea, vertigo, weakness, inflammation, etc. — are also the symptoms of disease. So-called disease is a process of resistance — resistance to poisons. It expels the cause of disease as surely as it expels calomel or ipecac. This fact is so very obvious, we are unable to understand why it cannot be grapsed by all.

Drugs are said to lose a degree of their potency by repetition. This does not express what actually takes place. It is not the drug that loses its potency. It is the body that loses power. The repeated use of a poison gradually overcomes or decreases vital resistance.

So long as it was believed that the symptoms following the taking of a poison represented drug action, it was legitimate to believe that when these symptoms no longer followed a dose of the poison, the drug had lost some of its potency. But when we realize that these symptoms are signs of vital resistance, that they are actions of the living body, we understand that the failure of these symptoms to follow a dose of the poison is due to a loss by the body of power to act.

This weakening of the powers of life, this subduing of the power of resistance, results in establishing what is called *toleration*. When toleration is established, that is, when the power of resistance is worn out, to produce the same effect — the same degree of resistance — the size of the dose must be progressively increased.

When medical men tell us that drugs lose their "remedial" effects by long continuance, we are to understand that *vital resistance* has been subdued. For the phenomena of *resistance* are what medical men mistakenly call the "remedial" effects of their drugs. They have not yet learned that it is the living body that acts (acts to expel the poison) and not the drug.

Toleration and lost resistance are one and the same thing. It is a matter of every day experience that as the body's power of resistance to a particular poison is reduced, it is less able to "react" to that poison.

The first effect of a toxin is always stimulation, which is merely another name for excitement or irritation. This is always followed by actions of the body (the so-called "reaction") to expel the poison. These actions (or "reactions") represent the process of resistance. The body refuses to tolerate the poison.

TOLERATION

When "stimulation" is frequently repeated, increasingly larger doses of the same poison or toxin are required to arouse a degree of intolerance that equals the intensity of the original "reaction." This lowered "reactive" power, this lessening of the defensive actions of the body, is called *toleration*.

Diminished resisting power (toleration) is a state of enervation. General enervation, however, produced — by drugs, excesses, by toxemia — diminishes resisting power to all poisons or excitants. This does not, in and of itself, represent a diminished susceptibility to the baneful influence of poisonous drugs. It may, however, represent, in addition to the increased enervation, a change in the methods of self-protection, a shifting from one method of defense to another and less expensive one — a passive resistance and a slow yielding to the influence of the poison.

This represents the cessation of active *resistance*, or partial submission to the poison. For submission, or lessened resistance, is what toleration really amounts to.

Passive resistance is doubtless accompanied with or accomplished by changes in the tissues, which, if not identical with those seen in the hands when these are subjected to repeated friction, are analogous to them. The hardening and thickening of the hands, that is the building up of callouses, is not the result of friction, but is a means of resisting friction. The tendency of friction is to wear away the skin, hence this must be continuously built up from beneath.

While the callous guards the underlying structures against the friction, it cripples all the powers of the skin. Such skin is not ideal — does not represent the physiological norm.

If you are not accustomed to using firey condiments and you undertake to use red pepper it causes the lips, mouth, tongue and throat to

—71—

burn intensely. When swallowed it produces discomfort in the stomach. There is later a feeling of discomfort in the intestine as the irritating pepper passes along. When, finally, it is expelled in the stools, the anus and rectum burn as much as did the mouth when the pepper was swallowed.

Persist in the use of the pepper and its irritating effect grows less and less until, finally, it produces no burning of the mouth and throat, no distress in the stomach and intestine, no burning of the rectum and anus. The membranes of the entire digestive tract become thickened and hardened in defense against the repeated irritation. The protective thickening impairs their other functions. The sense of taste is dulled, digestion is impaired. Doubtless something similar to this takes place in all the tissues of the body that are subjected to chronic irritation by alcohol, tobacco, caffeine, arsenic, opium, salt, and other poisons and irritants in common use. They, too, must undergo changes to defend themselves.

Adaptation to poisons, that is, the establishment of toleration, is accomplished by changes in the tissues that are away from the ideal and that cripple all the powers of the tissues.

I do not think it can be too strongly emphasized that adaptation to the use of a poison, that is, the establishment of *toleration*, is accomplished by a depravity of the organism. This fact was, so far as I know, first explained by Sylvester Graham more than a hundred years ago.

The greater the physiological depravity, the more of the poison will be "demanded" by the user and the more his body will tolerate without signs of active resistance. In others words, in precisely the proportion to which one becomes accustomed to the use of any poison is his system depraved and his defensive powers reduced. The ability to use large quantities of tobacco, for instance, without being made sick, instead of being an evidence of strength and physiological fitness, is an evidence of weakness and physiological depravity.

When tobacco is taken into the undepraved organism it is met with strong vital resistance. There follow in rapid succession distressing dizziness, muscular relaxation, tremor, weakness, perhaps fever, nausea, vomiting, diarrhea and, even, convulsions. Such a "reaction" always follows the introduction of tobacco into the undepraved organism; and the more vigorous and undepraved the organism the more prompt and powerful will be this "reaction."

It is only by commencing a career of depravity, with cautiously measured steps, that we may break down the body's resistance to the poison and, ultimately, bring about a condition in which the body seems actually to call for and embrace, as a friend, its arch foe.

The body may thus be so depraved that the deadliest poison may be habitually taken in considerable quantities and only result in an immediate feeling of apparent well being. Indeed, there may be, and usually is, much suffering if the depraved organism is denied the cause of its depravity.

The habitue may be able to take at one dose enough poison to kill six non-users. Arsenic may be used as freely as table salt, with as little immediate evidence of its poisonous character, once the body has been beaten into submission. Prussic acid, which kills like lightning, when the body is not accustomed to its use, may, by beginning with minute doses, and gradually using larger and larger doses, be used with considerable freedom as a means of "exhiliration" and intoxication.

The opium addict can take at one dose sufficient opium to kill several non-users outright. Instead of producing any immediate symptoms of poisoning in him, the opium results in an immediate feeling of well being. If he is denied his accustomed dose, he suffers intensely. Give him his accustomed poison and his sufferings vanish as if by magic. The cause of his suffering seems to cure his suffering — but only seems to, for the longer he uses the opium the more he suffers and the larger dose and the more frequent doses he will require to silence the outcries of his outraged system. The real effect of the dose is to re-narcotize his nerves, which can only cry out and reveal his true condition when they are no longer under the influence of the drug.

In the same way coffee will "cure" the headache it produces; tobacco will "steady" the nerves it has unsteadied; alcohol will "strengthen" the man it has weakened; "sleeping potions" cure the sleeplessness they have produced, only to make the sleeplessness worse and require a larger dose to "cure" next time. Stimulants weaken us by (apparently) making us stronger.

The ability of the carefully depraved organism to tolerate large doses of poisons and the fact of every day experience that the use of poisons by the physiologically depraved, instead of producing immediate symptoms of poisoning, results in the appearance and feeling of well-being, has led, even intelligent people, to stoutly deny the poisonous character of many poisons in habitual use. Because tobacco, or opium, or alcohol, or arsenic or coffee and tea, may be freely and habitually used without producing immediate death, or any of the distressing symptoms that indicate acute poisoning; but, on the contrary, so far as the feelings and actions of the users are concerned, they act as grateful "cordials", men and women are deceived by them. "My experience has shown that tobacco is very kind to me," says the tobacco user, while the opium addict informs us that his "experience has shown that opium is very kind to me."

Such "experience" is based, not alone on the deceptive appearances of drug-habituation, but is defective in that it forgets or ignores both the beginning and the end of the experience with the drug. If we accept the non-poisonous character of tea, coffee, tobacco, alcohol, opium, etc., on the basis of such "experience," we are forced to the fallacious conclusion that there is no such thing as a poison in nature. For there is no substance, however deadly, that the body cannot learn, by a career of physiological depravity, to tolerate.

The true test of the poisonous or non-poisonous character of any substance is its introduction into the undepraved — the intolerant — organism. By this test tobacco, alcohol, tea, coffee, opium, arsenic and all other drugs that are used for "exhiliration" and intoxication, are shown to be strongly anti-vital — poisonous.

The beginning of a poison vice is marked by evidences of acute poisoning. Thereafter, there are evidences of chronic poisoning. The end — no one disputes the end of opium addiction. Few today will deny the end of arsenic eating. Why close our eyes to the ends of alcoholism, nicotinism, caffeinism, etc.? Not until we include in our "experience" both the beginning and the end of a poison-vice are we justified in drawing conclusions from "our experience."

"Quick Relief"

Modern Medical Science has spawned its own myriads of charms and amulets. Yes, "science" has its own magic. Miracle and magic potencies are frequently discovered. After they are "tried and proven" at the bed side the patent medicine boys take over and the radios jam the air with high-pressure advertising as these boys sell their wares to all who can be induced to buy.

The patent medicine gang, unlike the "regular" practitioners, never sell "cures". They come as close to promising *cure* as they can without running afoul of the law. "Relief" is the big thing they promise. Relief, quick relief, from all your aches and pains — it is now the custom to promise relief only from "inorganic pains" — is the bait they dangle before the suckers.

How does this "quick relief" work? Here's an example. Some months ago I listened in on an *Alkaseltzer* program. A letter was read purporting to have come from a woman in a certain town in Illinois. She said she had been using alkaseltzer for five years. It gave her "relief" from headaches that other "remedies" had failed on. She also has an "acid stomach" and she had found it "no trick at all" to get "instant relief" with alkaseltzer.

For five years, according to her letter she has been "relieving" herself of her headaches and her "acid distress" with alkaseltzer. She is still using it for "relief". And she still *needs* the "relief". This is to say, she still suffers with headaches and abdominal distress. She has done nothing in this whole time to really remedy her troubles. Her contentment with temporary apparent relief has prevented her from seeking to know and remove the cause of her suffering. "Relief" is the chief obstacle between her and health.

The reading of her letter was followed by the song, "*Laugh Clown Laugh*". I thought it very appropriate. Although ignorance of the kind displayed by the letter is no laughing matter and clowning is out of place in health and disease, clowns and all others who have both a sense of humor and a saving amount of intelligence could not but laugh at her letter.

Alkaseltzer is a combination of aspirin (acetosalycilate) and common baking soda (sodium bicarbonate). The first sandbags the nerves into insensibility and damages the heart, the other temporarily neutralizes the acid in the stomach and interferes with digestion. Neither of them remove the cause of suffering.

Matching alkaseltzer in giving "amazing, quick relief" from "acid discomfort" are *Tums*. The radio pitch man advises: "Take Tums for quick relief" and follows up by saying "almost as soon as taken, Tums aid acid indigestion". I don't know why anybody should want to aid indigestion, but I am sure the makers of *Tums* know the secret.

Relief! relief!! relief!!! Thousands are yearly sacrificed on the altar of *relief*. They have pain and discomfort and they want "relief". Indeed, they are determined to have "relief" if they have to die to get it — and this is precisely what they do. They kill themselves "relieving" themselves of the consequences of their own indiscretions and follies. Give up their follies! Never! They are going to "enjoy" life. Cut out their indiscretions? Why should they? They "live" but once and they are going to have some "fun" .while they *live*.

Poor, purblind fools! Lured to their destruction by false pleasures and the promise of "quick relief". They go through life drugging themselves instead of ceasing the conduct that causes their suffering. They carry aspirin, alkaseltzer, tums and other "quick relief" pills in their purses, or buy them at the hot dog stands or the five and ten when they feel the "need" for them. They rush to the soda fountain and drink a glass of Bromo-seltzer for a headache or have a cup of coffee or a glass of coca-cola for the same condition. They "enjoy" the "cooling, refreshing" *relief* as it gurgles down their throats.

These various forms of "relief" do not merely encourage them to ignore the causes of their suffering and thus allow the suffering to grow greater; they, one and all, produce positive injury in their own right. They injure the digestive system, the nervous system, the heart, the kidneys, the blood, and other organs of the body. Each and everyone of them is enervating, hence, their use builds toxemia.

The more potent they are and the quicker they appear to relieve, the more enervating and damaging are they. The harm they actually do is commensurate with the good they appear to do. The larger the dose and the more frequent the doses, also, the more evil they are responsible for. There can be no true, no lasting, relief so long as they are used.

Some of them, like the caffeine of coffee, coca-cola and other cola drinks, are habit forming and these (also aspirin), produce worse pains than they appear to relieve. It were a thousand times better to clench your fist, grit your teeth and grin and bear your pain than to resort to these methods of gaining fictional relief.

If discomforts are not smothered, suppressed, by the "relief" measures, they will point to their origin and this may then be corrected. If pains are not "relieved" they will force the sufferer to cease the practices that produce them. Pain is a disciplinary measure. Destroy it, ignore its message, and you are sure for serious trouble. Somebody has said that the shortest road to a goal is often the foulest. In this case the apparent short road is really a short-cut to the cemetery. Heed the message of pain and you will save yourself much future difficulty. "The wise will understand".

The "relief" system is an arch deceiver. It leads its dupes to believe they are doing something constructive. So long as they are "comfortable" they think they are well. They are taught by the "relief" mongers to believe that the methods that "relieve" them actually help them.

The "relief" system kills. The poor asthmatic feels that he is helped, even that his life is saved, by the shot of adrenalin or by the smoke of burning stramonium leaves. He does not realize that each dose of these "reliefs" fastens the asthma habit upon him and prevents recovery. Headache sufferers turn to "relief". Those who have constipation seek "relief". Everywhere "relief" is what is sought. Nowhere is it sought to remove cause.

The medical profession is responsible for this eternal seeking after "relief". This profession has taught mankind to seek for and be content with fictional "relief". This profession devotes itself almost exclusively to supplying "relief". It never seeks to find and remove causes. It has led the race off on the "relief" tangent and further away from the paths of truth and nature. The patent medicine trade is a legitimate offshoot of the regular drug trade. Always it is a faithful reflection of the medical practice of the time.

GETTING WELL

The death of the patent medicine industry will be followed immediately by the death of the regular drug trade. Physicians and patent medicine vendors are siamese twins. They cannot be severed without the death of both of them.

The Cry of the Distressed

Out over the nation in December there went an anguished cry for help. Over all the country side it reverberated. Over the highways and down the country lanes it floated. Over hills and through the valleys the sound was heard. It echoed and reechoed throughout the cities. "We need your help. Desperately," came the anguished cry.

The voice was the voice of Jeannie Cameron, the words were the words of the millions who suffer with arthritis. The vehicle that carried the plea for help was the December issue of the *Coronet*. "We have submitted to all known treatments," says Miss Cameron, herself a sufferer with arthritis and an inmate of a sanitarium devoted to the care of arthritis patients out on the New Mexico desert, "and have stubbornly refused to respond."

This is the despairing cry, not merely of Miss Cameron, who has suffered for years, but of all others who so suffer. Hopelessness is their lot and so-called medical science is as helpless to do anything for them as they, themselves, are to get around without their canes, crutches and wheel chairs.

They do a lot of whistling in the dark. It helps to keep up their courage. "We are not pessimistic," says Miss Cameron, "we are waiting, still hopefully, for that 'somebody' who will one day discover the secret, and release us from our bonds." Hoping, vainly hoping, for a saviour longing for the time to come when some magic remedy will be found that will give them health, they manage to keep up their courage while watching themselves grow gradually worse.

She tells about some of her fellow-sufferers at the sanitarium. For instance, there is pretty red-haired Barbara who is only 23. She had her first "attack" of arthritis back in Michigan when she was only 13. Miss Cameron tells us: "She went through the various clinics in the Middle West before coming out here. She had all the treatments: fever therapy, transfusions, huge doses of vitamin D, shots of all kinds, injections of gold. Each thing helps, temporarily. Then it wears off and that particular treatment, when tried again, has no effect. On crutches, by strength of will alone, Barbara finished high school. Then she gave in and went to bed, practically for keeps. When I first came she got into her wheel-chair for about an hour in the morning and again in the afternoon. Twice a day she walked half way down the hall and back, perhaps 20 steps each way — with her crutches, of course. The rest of the time she spent in bed.

"Eight months later, Barbara is still doing just that."

This is a sad story — a story of ten years of needless suffering by a little girl who might now be enjoying life and serving the community in which she lives. It is a story that can be duplicated thousands of times in the sanitariums, hospitals, clinics and nursing homes of the country. It is more than the story of the sufferings of a little girl — it is the story of the failure of *medical science*.

"Cathy was a perfectly normal American girl —and a freshman in college. She danced, she swam, she played tennis, she made good grades," and, then, she developed arthritis. Her story is not recounted, but we can assume that it does not greatly differ from that of Barbara. She probably "got the works." Everything was done for her "that science can do."

Now "Cathy has casts for her legs and spends several hours a day lying in bed with them on. They are tiring and wretchedly hot. After she rests for six weeks perhaps, all the swelling in her knees goes down. Then with her crutches she walks, three steps. Then six. Then ten. Down to my room and back, slowly and carefully.

"And then, one night we hear her crying pitifully and in the morning via the grape vine, the whole corridor knows. Cathy is off her feet again, back in the casts, the pain and soreness almost more than she can take."

Blasted hopes more unbearable than the physical pain! Yesterday, high hope; this morning, black despair. Such is the experience of arthritis sufferers under medical abuse. Cathy's story is an old one. There are thousands of Cathys all over America today.

Tom, she says "has had all the various treatments" including an "exceedingly painful" and "not particularly satisfactory" operation of breaking adhesions. He "has been out of circulation now for almost four years." Miss Cameron thinks he is "*better*" now — the italics are hers. "He *was* in bed all day two years ago. Now he sits out in the yard a couple of hours each afternoon."

How soon after she wrote this Tom was heard "crying pitifully" and the whole corridor learned via the grapevine that Tom is back in bed again, we will not know. These cases have their "ups" and "downs" — they grow worse and they appear to grow better, but there is a steady relentless progress of the pathology.

Miss Cameron well describes the progressiveness of the pathology as follows: "We have always felt well. Full of pep with energy to spare. Then suddenly we realize that for the past three months we have tired easily. Our feet begin to hurt; we take extra shoes to the office. Our hands are swollen and sore; we wince when enthusiastic salesmen give us the old friendly grip. One day we lean pensively on our elbows, and are brought out of our dreamy mood with a bang. Those elbows, too, hurt frightfully. In my case I dragged back and forth to the office for a full year —and by that time my hands and feet were badly crippled, my knees stiff, my hair gray."

From this stage the condition goes on — joint after joint becomes swollen, painful, stiff, finally, ankylosed. From dragging back and forth unassisted they drag back and forth with a cane, then with crutches, then are pushed around in a wheel chair. At first they can get out of bed and dress themselves. They can wash themselves, take their own baths and comb their own hair. But, after a time, they have to be helped in and out of bed, an attendant must wash and bathe them and comb their hair, even feed them. They have to be lifted from bed to chair and from chair to bed.

Their teeth are pulled, their tonsils are removed, their gall bladders extirpated, their appendices cut out, their ovaries and seminal vesicles excised. their sinuses are drained or chiselled out; they are given colonic irrigations, autogeneous vaccines, other vaccines, gold salts, vitamin D, "fever" therapy, blood plasma, hot baths, mineral baths, massage, salicylates, and a host of other forms of abuse.

None of their physicians ever think of so simple and so rational, even if not "scientific", a plan as removing the cause of their suffering. They are treated and treated and, finally, sent away to a magic climate. The dry climate of the desert is supposed to be good for them. The climate doesn't work any better than the treatment and death alone ends their suffering.

Miss Cameron says: "we seem to live forever, dragging on for years and years, exhausting the patience and finances of our families. We seldom die of this (arthritis). When something else does the trick, our epitaph is invariably the same: 'Well, really — after all, it's a blessing.'"

Painful and imprisoned existence is a long-drawn out existence, even if it is a short one. The old saying about married men that "they don't live longer, it only seems longer," is appropriate here. Arthritis sufferers don't live forever; it only seems forever. Their days are long periods of waiting for night; their nights long periods of anguished waiting for day.

Hope alternates with despair; a brief period of ease with a period of suffering. There comes a brief period of apparent improvement only to be followed by greater suffering and an increase in their trouble.

"We can wake up of a morning feeling rested and without a pain," says Miss Cameron. "Surely, a miracle has happened. But when we try to rise, to step, the very minute those wasted muscles, which are always the heritage of arthritis, are called upon to do their part, the dream is over. The pain and stiffness are there and within an hour or two, the rested feeling is a thing of the past.

"We move about, yes, but as though hampered by chains, and with balls of lead attached to our ankles. We live, but as though we are under some strange hypnotic spell."

These poor sufferers have our sympathies. We have watched them suffer and we have seen them grow worse and worse. We have seen them die. We can, in our imaginations, place ourselves in their positions and realize their hopelessness and despair.

But to us the most tragic part of these cases is their refusal to accept a tried and proven way out of their suffering. Year after year, as thousands of new cases develop, they go through the treatments mentioned above and go through the same painful road to helpless and hopeless invalidism. They, one and all (or nearly all), try the old failures; hoping against hope, that, although they have failed to help millions of others, "maybe they will somehow help me."

This year thousands of new cases of arthritis will develop in America. They will go through the clinics and hospitals. "Foci of infection" will be removed, shots will be given, gold salts will be administered, "fever" therapy will be given them, they will be given huge doses of vitamin D, they will be massaged and bathed and drugged. And, they will end up in two to four years like Barbara, Cathy, Tom and Miss Cameron have ended.

Year after year this process has gone on; year after year it will continue. Only a few, a very few, will forsake this folly and accept a rational plan of care and get well. All cases of arthritis can make a speedy and permanent recovery if they are given proper care at the start. None of them need ever become invalids. Even after they have suffered for months and years most of them can get well and be restored to usefulness. It is their tragedy that they go on hoping for a magic remedy that will restore them to health and reject a sane plan of care.

Miss Cameron pleads with doctors (she means physicians), scientists and philanthropists to "take us into your family and work hard for us." She is willing to beg, buy or steal a *cure*. She is not willing to earn it. She wants vicarious salvation. Her experience with *cures*, her observations of *cures* when used on others, have not served to open her eyes.

She says of the patients in the sanitarium where she is: "Most of these people are young. They are as valiant as they come, consistently optimistic, and they have all tried — tried so hard. But they will have to wait, it seems, until something new is discovered."

How tragically sad that these young people, after all their trying of all the *cures* are content to sit around and wait — wait hopefully, optimistically — until a new *cure* is discovered! They are waiting, just waiting, for a new drug, a new vaccine, a new vitamin, a new bath, a new fever machine, a new voodoo trick of one kind or another, so they can *try* this, also.

Miss Cameron pleads for money for research. "Little is being contributed to our aid," she laments. *"For every dollar spent on research for us, four hundred dollars are spent on work done for tuberculosis. • • • * Millions for the care of infantile paralysis, cancer, diabetes and all the others." Don't forget us arthritics, you who endow research and hospitals for incurables, she pleads.

And yet, is it not obvious for all who have eyes to see, that all of this vast amount of money spent on "research" is wasted? Where is the cure for tuberculosis? for infantile paralysis? for cancer? Millions have been spent in "researching" for the cause and cure of colds. Where is the *cure;* what is the cause?

"Research" offers arthritics no hope. It will not discover the cause of arthritis. It will find no cure therefor. The "research" boys will pay themselves handsome salaries out of the endowment funds, they will torture thousands of helpless animals, try out new drugs and vaccines on arthritics, issue learned reports of their work and assure us that they are just on the verge of discovering the cause and cure. They only need another hundred millions dollars to enable them to make the discovery.

Everywhere we turn, the "researchers" are empty handed. There is much blood — the blood of innocent victims — upon their hands, but there is nothing of value to justify giving them more millions with which to perpetrate more of their ghastly experiments. The death of no number of animals upon the cross of vivisection can buy salvation for Man. There is no vicarious atonement.

Nor is endowing hospitals for the care of "incurables" the remedy. This gives the "incurables" a place to stay and a feeling of security, it provides jobs for parasitic physicians and nurses, but it "makes no brick". Health does not come out of such places. The "incurables" that go into them remain "incurables." Too many of them would rather malinger in such institutions than get well.

It is time for us to realize that responsibility for recovery rests squarely upon the shoulders of the sick person and that no one else can assume that responsibility. Those who reject a sane way of life and a rational plan of care and prefer the voodoo tricks of the modern shaman must pay for their folly.

In the words of an ancient law-giver: "Behold, this day I have placed before you life and death, blessings (health) and curses (disease); choose life that ye may live."

Killing Our Children

The more I see of women's magazines, the better I understand why so many women buy *Esquire*. (The more I see of *Esquire*, the more I wonder why anybody ever reads any magazine.) Women's magazines seem to have two chief purposes — namely (1) to sell clothes, cosmetics, baby foods, etc., and (2) to carry medical propaganda. An occasional article on how to catch and hold a husband only serves as spice for their monotonous diet of cosmetics, fur coats and medical hokum.

_ _ *McCalls* for Nov. 1943 carries an article by Philip Moen Stimson, M. D., entitled "RHEUMATIC FEVER—Deadliest Enemy of Childhood." It is an unusual article for a medical man to write. These men usually require several thousand words in which to tell us that they don't know, but Stimson can say "We don't know" in about a thousand words.

From the article we learn that rheumatic fever "kills more children between the ages of 5 and 15 than any other disease." *Killing* "4 times as many as diphtheria, measles, scarlet fever, whooping cough, infantile paralysis, epidemic meningitis combined." It "leaves many survivors with damaged hearts" and "is responsible for a million individuals with heart disease in this country today."

We learn something else that should be of interest to our readers: this is that *rheumatic fever* is not the clean-cut, specific disease that the physician can diagnose with ease. It is not the "great imitator" that "syphilis" is, but it does some imitating itself.

It may manifest itself as swollen joints (arthritis), or as chorea (St. Vitus dance), or as nodules under the skin, or as "certain skin eruptions" and "more rarely, as abdominal pain." Stimson says "this is a tricky fifth-column disease that strikes different children in different ways. Instead of attacking openly, it may employ any of a number of different disguises."

This old demon does not fight fair. He makes *sneak attacks* on our children and fools our physicians who, thanks be to Heaven, are always on guard to protect us and our children from the powers of darkness. Except for these guardians no doubt other demons would be as deadly as this cowardly underhanded devil that dons different disguises in order to slip through our guards and get at us.

When are medical men going to abandon this old voodooistic conception of disease and cease using language and terms reminiscent of it? When are they going to stop talking of *disease* as though it were an entity, an organism of some kind, that attacks us without provocation and strikes in the dark because of the utter malignancy of its heart?

After naming the above different "commonest of its (rheumatic fever) strange manifestations", Stimson says: "some of these symptoms may be due to other causes than rheumatic fever." Is rheumatic fever the cause, or is it the "disease"? Does the rheumatic fever produce the symptoms, or do the symptoms and the pathology behind them constitute the rheumatic fever? Which is cause and which is effect?

If the rheumatic fever is the cause, what is rheumatic fever? Where does it come from and where does it go? If it is the demon that "strikes"

children and "employs a number of different disguises" where does it hide out when not attacking the children? Can we trace it to its lair and
kill it in some way?

Rheumatic fever is merely a name — a name
given to a variable group of symptoms It is not
an entity. It never strikes, it never dons any disguises, it never does anything .

"Someday we hope to know the exact cause
of rheumatic fever", says Stimson. They don't
know its cause — not, even, its inexact cause — at
the present time. But why talk about the rheumatic fever being the cause of "these symptoms"
and then talk of rheumatic fever as though it is
the effect, not the cause? Why? Because voodooism distorts all of their reasoning.

The cause of rheumatic fever is not known,
but they think they "have some strong clues."
The *hemolytic streptococcus* (a bacteria) "seems
to be 'one of the responsible agents'". But these
little fellows who have been given a bad name
don't seem to be the real cause. Instead their
action "may be likened to a detonator which sets
off a stick of dynamite or a bomb." These
malicious little devils seem to derive a certain
fiendish glee out of pulling the trigger of an
already loaded gun and watching the explosion.
They are not the *dynamite*, they are only the
spark that sets it off.

. What is the dynamite? What loads the bomb?
What loads the gun? What prepares the charge
for the explosion? Or to abandon metaphor, which
only serves to conceal ignorance, what is the
primary, the basic, cause of rheumatic fever?

Echo answers: "What is the primary, the
basic, cause of rheumatic fever?

Stimson can only reply: "Someday we hope
to know the exact cause of rheumatic fever."

They'll never learn its cause while chasing elusive Jack-O-Lanterns over the swamps and bogs of voodooism.

If they don't know its cause, what can they do about it? Stimson answers "much of this suffering could be avoided — if the symptoms are recognized early and treatment begun at once."

To begin treatment means to begin dosing the patient with poisonous drugs. It does not mean to begin to remove an unknown cause. It means suppressing symptoms. It means "plenty of good nourishing foods to keep up your strength." It means autogeneous vaccines, and sulfa drugs. It means opium, salicylates, ice bags and a lot of other destructive, enervating and, often, fatal measures. These are the things that kill and cripple the children.

No wonder Stimson says these children must stay in bed six months! It is not a wonder that so many die; the wonder is that as many survive as do. Stimson says they must spend these months in bed "under expert medical and nursing care" and adds that "as a rule this can best be obtained in a hospital."

After the children come out of the hospital, providing they come out alive, those "children whose hearts are too badly damaged to permit this (to return to school) may in some cities attend 'cardiac classes' where school work goes along on a special schedule which includes naps' and fresh air. Others may study at home and be provided with a home teacher."

If you live in a city where the "cardiac classes" are not held and do not have the money with which to provide your child with a "home teacher," you need not worry about your child growing up in ignorance, because he "will die before the age of thirty-five." For such a short life of invalidism, an education does not mean much.

Stimson tells us how to prevent rheumatic fever in our children. It is this: "the mother should do everything possible to keep her child from having colds and sore throats."

Its as simple as that. Don't let your child have colds. How? Ah! This is so simple! You just "keep your child dry, warm and at a distance from everybody who has a cold or any infection whatsoever." All of this will be easy if you rear the child as a hermit out on a desert and keep him under a glass bowl that is constantly bathed in formaldehyde, and keep a Bunsen burner always burning under his nose.

Don't let your child have sore throats, "for we know that frequently a child 'comes down' with rheumatic fever within a short time after he has had tonsillitis, scarlet fever or a 'streptococcus sore throat'," and that "rheumatic fever is at its peak in the late winter and early spring when sore throats are prevalent."

How do you prevent your child from having sore throats, you ask? Oh! That's all very simple! You just keep your child locked up in the attic so that he will not come in contact with anyone who has sore throats or "infections" of any kind. This should be easy.

But, "if by some mischance your child does contract rheumatic fever, the outlook need not be so hopeless." You can send him to the hospital for six months, to the "cardiac classes" for a few years, or have him taught at home, and bury him early. One other precaution must be emphasized. It is this: "Every child who has ever had the disease" (rheumatic fever) "needs constant but unobstrusive watching by a physician to prevent, if possible, any recurrence. For it is the subsequent attacks to which the child is liable up to adolescence, and sometimes after, which damage an already damaged heart.

Redoubled efforts must be made to keep the child from catching colds and sore throats; for any streptococcus infection may be instrumental in again activating rheumatic fever."

All this adds up to the fact that you should move to a larger desert, use more formaldehyde and get a larger Bunsen burner or confine your child in a smaller attic. Only thus can you re-double your efforts to keep your child from contacting other people among whom many at all times have sore throats, colds, tonsillitis and other "infections." You must, by all means keep your child from "catching" colds and sore throats. Teach him not to *catch* everything he sees. To *catch* things is simply not good form.

Stimson's article is conspicuous for one thing — he does not advise the removal of the tonsils. I don't mean that he says this is inadvisable. He merely does not say anything about it. Ten years ago the advice to "have the child's ton-sils removed" would have consumed the greater part of the article. Medical authorities now tell us that the concensus of opinion of unpreju-diced students of the matter is that until some-one produces incontrovertable evidence that children without tonsils are definitely protected against rheumatism, routine removal of the ton-sils is not justifiable.

One leading medical authority, after admit-ting ignorance of the cause of rheumatic fever, says that the "modern concept" of the causative role played by "streptococcal infections" gives them a "more rational attitude," towards the effects of removing the tonsils in preventing rheumatic fever. He adds that while removal of the tonsils "may" diminish the chance of acquiring an "infection," the "very fact that a very slight streptococcal infection of the naso-pharynx may induce a rheumatic occurrence shows how ineffective" removal of the tonsils may be in this respect. He points out, also that after the tonsils (the faucial tonsils) are removed "much lymphoid tissue is left in the naso and oropharynx" and this may "harbor streptococi."

The fact is that there remains in the throat, after the tonsils are removed, far more lymphoid tissue than is removed. Therefore, if removal of lymphoid tissue is the way to prevent rheumatic fever, it would be necessary to remove all that exists in the throat and adjacent structures. Even if this were possible and resulted in no other evil, it would ruin the throat.

Disease can never be prevented by vandalizing the body. Destroying organs and parts is a fool's plan of prevention. We told this to the medical, surgical and dental professions years ago, but they were too deeply narcotized with the sweet essence of self-conceit and so puffed up with their arrogant assumption that they, and they alone know anything about the body and its "diseases" they refused to listen. The public, too, refused to listen the public paid, paid through the nose (and throat) for its blindness and stupidity. The medical, surgical and dental gangsters were well paid for their arrogance and their haughty pose as infallible near-gods. Now that their self-made pedestals are crumbling, I imagine I can hear them asking: "Where do we go from here?"

"Curing" Arthritis

An item in the *Townsend National Weekly* for May 15, tells us that physicians are still seeking a "cure" for arthritis, of which there are more than 7,000,000 cases in the United States, alone. The item says: "The toll of arthritis, according to the U. S. Public Health Service, accounted for 300,000,000 man-hours lost on the production line last year."

The item also tells us that "only a small proportion can hope for a definite and complete recovery." The medical profession is now engaged in a "long-range enquiry as to the nature and cause of arthritis, one of the 'mystery' diseases of modern medicine." Then we learn that the "disease" is very old, that "it crippled dinosaurs of the Triassic period" and "even laid up the cave bear."

We don't know why, but the item adds, "obviously some progress should have been made." The mere fact that a "disease" is very old does not render "progress" obviously expected. The profession cannot make progress for the reason that the false principles upon which it works are as old as the "disease." The item adds: "But very little is on the credit side for all the investigation."

A picture of modern (?) "medicine" as it approaches this old problem in a very old way is contained in these words of the news item: "Treating arthritis with gold salts has produced some good results, but the medical profession is not yet satisfied with it as a general method.

In earlier stages, it has resulted in improvement in 78 percent of cases."

Does the profession have any method of treating any so-called "disease" with which it is *satisfied?* Does is possess a single method of treatment that is sufficiently satisfactorv that it is not searching for another method to take its place? If so it has not seen fit to reveal this fact to the public.

Why is it not "satisfied" with its methods of treatment? Simply because they are not effective, they do not cure. They do not work because they do not remove cause.

What have gold salts to do with the cause of arthritis? Nothing. Are they given to remove the cause of arthritis? No. The medical profession does not even know the cause of arthritis. They cannot remove a cause of which they are profoundly ignorant. The claim that these salts produce improvement in 78 per cent of cases when employed in early stages is hot air. If they do not remove cause they cannot produce improvement. If they remove cause they would not merely produce improvement, they would produce complete recovery.

The use of gold salts in arthritis is merely another of "medicine's" spectacular methods of palliation. It is part of their system (?) of voodooism. Gold salts are poisonous and injurious and their use is not without damage to the patient.

Finally, the news item tells us: "The most effective treatment is confined to rest in bed for several months; proper diet; the removal, perhaps, of some local infection — such as bad teeth, etc.; and exercise in warm water pools, massage, etc."

If this is the "most effective treatment", what, in Heaven's name, is the "least effective" treatment? This is the popular and most used form of treatment, the treatment employed by most of the 7,000,000 patients now suffering with arthritis in this country. This is the kind of treatment that causes them to say: "only a small proportion can hope for definite and complete recovery." And this treatment does not produce the recovery in these few cases.

All over America thousands upon thousands of people are undergoing this "most effective treatment" and are going from bad to worse. Joint after joint is being involved under this treatment. Ankylosis follows deformity. Patient after patient becomes a hopelessly bed-ridden invalid.

Removing tonsils, pulling teeth, cutting out gall bladders, removing appendices, extirpating ovaries, excising seminal vesicles, draining and chiseling out sinuses, and all the other voodooism that pretends to remove "foci of infection" is not remedying arthritis. Operation after operation upon the same patient, the patient growing progressively worse, should prove to even the die-hards in the surgical camp, that removing "foci of infection" is a delusion.

The warm pools of the country are crowded with arthritis sufferers. They go back time after time to bathe and swim in these warm waters. But they do not get well. After a few trips to these resorts, the arthritis sufferer becomes so badly crippled up he can no longer swim in them.

Proper diet! What is proper diet? The diets fed these patients are certainly not proper. These patients continue to grow worse on these "proper diets." They become hopeless cripples on such diets.

Rest in bed! How can they rest when plied with drugs, given massages and taken out for swims? What is rest? Does the "medical" profession even know the meaning of the term?

Rest in bed for several months! Why several months? If these cases are properly cared for from the start, they should be fully well in three to six weeks. The failure of this whole program is seen in its demand for "rest in bed for several months."

Massage! What can massage do? It can palliate symptoms. It can slow up the stiffening of joints. It can't remove cause. It can't restore health. It is not necessary if the patient is properly cared for.

While taking the whole of the above described "most effective treatment", these patients continue to grow from bad to worse. It was the failure of this plan of care that caused the medical profession to try gold salts. It is the failure of this form of treatment that permits thousands of sufferers to become hopeless invalids every year. It is the failure of this form of care that causes them to say: "only a small proportion can hope for a definite and complete recovery." They are still seeking a *cure* for arthritis. Why? Because this "most effective treatment" is only effective in making these patients worse.

The experienced observer knows that arthritis starts usually in one joint, at most, two joints, and after a variable period spreads to other joints. Joint after joint becomes involved, until, in many cases, every movable joint in the body is involved.

The joints are painful, swollen, deformed, stiff, and, finally, grow together — *ankylose* — so that they become permanently destroyed. The patient, or parts of the body, become fixed in

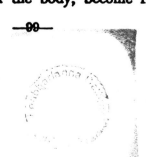

awkward, strained and deformed positions, long before he becomes completely helpless. First a cane, then crutches and, later, a wheel chair are his means of locomotion. Often he is carried from bed to chair and from chair to bed for years before death finally brings his suffering and helplessness to an end.

If he goes to a physician when his trouble first develops, he is likely to have a number of operations plus all the treatments in the books before he begins to realize that the physicians know no more about what should be done than he does. He will spend years of time and a small fortune in money in his effort to get well and all the while, he will see his condition grow progressively worse. He will travel from physician to physician, from surgeon to surgeon, from hospital to hospital, from sanitarium to sanitarium, from spa to spa, from climate to climate.

It is all so futile. He may realize this too late or he may have his eyes opened before the pathological changes in his joints have gone beyond redemption. He may dose himself with salicylates, under the physician's directions of course, until this wrecks his heart. His pain is great and he wants the "relief" these drugs afford, even if, in the end, they do kill him. He will do all of these things and not get well — he will, on the contrary, grow from bad to worse.

Every treatment that ignores cause, that fails to remove cause, permits the patient to grow worse. The above "most effective treatment" does not remove cause but does produce enervation. It is criminal treatment and every physician who so treats a patient and accepts money therefor is obtaining money under false pretenses.

Such treatment will some day be generally recognized as malpractice. It is a very bad form

of abusing the sick. Its total failure is testified
to by the millions of sufferers with arthritis
who have undergone months and years of this
"most effective treatment" and grown from bad
to worse thereunder. Only the ignorant and
credulous can be induced to submit to it. Only
commercialism keeps physicians employing it.

Arthritis is due to toxemia in a gouty subject.
By a gouty subject is meant one with the gouty
diathesis. The gouty diathesis is not the cause
of arthritis. Toxemia is the cause of this "disease."

Toxemia is due to inhibition of excretion —
is the result of retention of metabolic waste
and decomposition products absorbed from the
digestive tract, due to checking of secretion
and excretion.

Secretion and excretion are inhibited by enervation and this, in turn, is due to a mode of living that expends nerve energy and causes enervation. Enervation impairs elimination (inhibits
excretion and secretion in general). Toxins are
retained, producing toxemia. Toxins, in turn,
overstimulate, resulting in further enervation.
Chronic poisoning results.

Chronic poisoning establishes toleration by
breaking down resistance to its influence. Toleration is a state of passive resistance.

Toxemic saturation is a state of toxemia
slightly below the point of active resistance. This
point, obviously, must vary from the low level
of toxic toleration established by the vigorous
and healthy to the high toxic toleration established by the weak and chronically toxemic.

When the toxemic state has reached the saturation point? all that is needed to bring on a crisis — an acute disease — is exposure, worry, fear,
overwork, or just one more depression of any
kind to give an added check to elimination and
push the toxemia above the point of toleration.

In gouty subjects the resulting so-called "disease" is likely to be arthritis or some other form of so-called *rheumatic* "disease."

The remedy for arthritis is physical, mental and physiological rest until toxemia is eliminated and nerve energy *is* restored and, thereafter, a mode of living that does not produce enervation. Arthritis rapidly ceases when proper care is instituted from the start. Rapid recoveries often follow even at later stages. The deformity may be allowed to reach a stage where it cannot be overcome. Only pain and inflammation can be ended in these cases. We venture to estimate that more than three-fourths of the more than 7,000,000 cases of arthritis now in this country can recover full health. Most of them could attain good health in three months or less.

Endocarditis

The heart is a hollow, conical, muscular organ. The Greek word for heart is *Kardia;* the Greek word for muscle is *Mys*. Accordingly, the heart muscle is known as the *myocardium*. The cavities of the heart are lined with a thin serous membrane known as the endocardium. The heart is invested by a thin serous membrane known as the *pericardium*.

Itis, as we have repeatedly emphasized in these pages, is a little Greek word used to designate inflammation. When it is attached to the end of the name of an organ or part of the body, it signifies inflammation in that organ or part. Hence:

Myocarditis is inflammation of the heart muscle.

Endocarditis is inflammation of the lining membrane of the heart.

Pericarditis is inflammation of the investing membrane of the heart.

Endomyocarditis is inflammation of both the lining (endocardium) and muscle (myocardium) of the heart.

Endopericarditis is inflammation of the lining membrane of the heart "complicated" by inflammation of its investing membrane (pericardium).

Endoperimyocarditis is inflammation of the endocardium, pericardium and myocardium.

If it is all clear to you that each of these fifteen dollar words means that some part or parts of the heart is inflamed, you know as much as your physician about the matter. You already know that inflammation is a great excess of blood in a circumscribed area of the body giving rise to heat, redness, swelling, pain and disturbed function. You already know that inflammation in one organ or part of the body is the same as inflammation in another organ or part. Also you already know that the differences in the symptoms produced by inflammation in one organ and those produced by inflammation in another organ, are not due to any differences in the inflammation, but to differences in the functions of the organs.

Inflammation of the tongue will interfere with chewing, talking and swallowing; inflammation of the heart interferes with heart action. The symptoms differ because the structures and functions of the organs differ. The inflammation is the same; the cause may also be the same.

Several varieties of *endocarditis* are listed in the nosologies. These are:

Chronic, which is chronic inflammation.

Exudative, which is acute inflammation.

Malignant, which is considered to be usually secondary to a suppurative ulceration elsewhere in the body.

Ulcerative, in which there is necrosis or ulceration of the valves of the heart.

Now, the differences between acute and chronic inflammation are those of degree and duration. The differences between acute and chronic inflammation in the heart are the same as the differences between acute and chronic inflammation in the tonsils, stomach, kidneys. The differences between simple inflammation of the heart and ulceration of the heart are the same as those between ordinary catarrhal inflammation of the nose and ulceration of the nose; the same as those between gastritis and gastric ulcer; the same as those between mucus colitis and ulcerative colitis. The ulceration is merely another step or stage in the progressive development of pathology.

If this is all clear to you, you know more about these heart "diseases" than your physician; for he thinks of each of these conditions as distinct "diseases," or *entities*, and thinks that each one of them is not only caused by a different cause, but that they are the result of causes different from those that produce inflammation elsewhere in the body. This last part is not entirely correct, for he does think some heart "disease" is caused by "rheumatism," "gonorrhea", "syphilis", and "germs". Beyond this he hardly has an idea about the cause of heart "disease."

Both acute and chronic "diseases" are divided into *benign* and *malignant*.

The *malignant* types of acute "disease" are made malignant by absorption of putrescent infection arising from decomposition .of animal foods in the stomach and bowels.

The chronic types of "disease" are made malignant by putresence arising from degeneration (oxygen starvation) within the morbid growth or tissue itself.

Malignant endocarditis results from pus absorption from suppurative processes elsewhere in the body or from an overwhelming putresence arising in the digestive tract. Gonorrhea is said to often cause it. If this is so, the gonorrheal patient must be badly abused by treatment.

Endocarditis is usually confined to the valves of the heart and should be called valvular endocarditis, or by the older term *valoulitis*.

I will not discuss the symptoms of endocarditis, for the condition cannot be diagnosed by the symptoms alone and the layman should not attempt self-diagnosis in conditions of the heart.

Indeed, I find too much worry and anxiety over the heart. All kinds of symptoms that are felt in the region of the heart, but, which, in most cases, have no relation to the heart, are causes of much fear and apprehension.

It will be more profitable if we discuss the causes of endocarditis, for if the causes are known these may be avoided. If they are not known, a knowledge that you have endocarditis is a cause of worry only.

I have already hinted that endocarditis is caused by the same causes that produce other so-called "diseases." In discussing this fact, I shall quote from the section on endocarditis in Vol. 7 of *The Hygienic System*. There I say:

"Acute endocarditis is a symptomatic affection and is always found in conjunction with other affections. It is the custom to credit rheumatism, tonsilitis, etc., as causes. These affections cause nothing, but are antecedent, concomitant and successive effects of the same toxic state that causes the heart affection. Years of over eating and plethory with the autotoxemic state resulting from absorption of toxins from the intestines produces both the rheumatism and the endocarditis. The rheumatism may be severe, or it may be so mild that the patient does not go to bed. It seldom leaves the heart unaffected. Indeed, the heart is subject to toxin-infection continuously and it is possible for valvular endocarditis to develop without other rheumatic development.

"Tobacco strikes hard at the heart and blood vessels as well as at the nervous system, liver and kidneys. The use of tobacco increases the pulse rate from five to ten beats a minute, and in the case of the man who is continually smoking, the increase of the rate becomes permanent. The increased pulse rate is accompanied by a small increase in blood pressure, which sets in a few minutes after smoking is started and persists until the smoking ceases. That the heart of even "moderate" smokers is less efficient under strain is well known to athletes and trainers.

"Malignant endocarditis is never primary, but results from pus infection from peritonitis, pus absorption, septic infection, etc. * * *

"Chronic endocarditis may follow one or more crises of acute endocarditis, or it may start as a mild inflammation or degeneration that is not noticeable until extensive changes have occurred. It is never primary, but develops as a part of the general pathology of the body. Alcoholism, lead poisoning, tobacco and chronic nephritis (inflammation of the kidney) favor its development."

The use of the salicylates in rheumatism also leads to heart disease. These drugs are given to "relieve" pain only, and are not claimed to have any curative value. No doubt their use is one of the chief reasons for endocarditis developing as a complication of acute and, even, chronic rheumatism.

The cause of causes, the cause that lies back of the rheumatism, back of the peritonitis, back of the septic infection, etc., is toxemia resulting from retention of body waste. Lowered nerve energy checks elimination producing toxemia. Lowered nerve energy (enervation) results from the thousand-and-one things in our mode of living that collectively use up nerve energy in excess. The final, or remote, cause of endocarditis is a wrong mode of living.

It is generally held, that while acute simple arthritis is rarely fatal, it rarely leaves the heart valves undamaged. It seems to me that whether or not the valves are left damaged depends upon the severity of inflammation and the kind of care the patient receives. The valves are probably left undamaged much more often than we are aware of; or the damage may often be so slight as to be. negligible.

Where the damage is marked so that the function of the heart is crippled, compensatory enlargement of the heart follows under favorable conditions and *good health* may be preserved for many years. Such an incurably crippled heart can be greatly relieved by a life of moderation and frugal eating. With such care in living, nature will tolerate the condition and often the heart will be able to carry on for many years.

Malignant endocarditis is very frequently fatal and where not fatal there is usually more or less permanent damage to the heart.

Many cases of chronic endocarditis are pronounced *incurable* only because drugs do not *cure* them. Recovery in these cases often follows removal of cause plus rest.

I do not advise heart sufferers to attempt to care for themselves, therefore, any detailed discussion of care in these cases would be out of place here. In general the care may be said to consist of two processes:

1. It is necessary to correct nutrition by correcting the mode of living and by fasting and rest, eliminate toxemia and restore nerve energy.

2. All sources of infection must be removed. Abcesses must be drained, gastrointestinal decomposition must be corrected and proper drainage of the pelvis re-established where this is faulty.

All medical authorities are agreed that the most important factor in the treatment of acute myocarditis is rest. In fact they are so determined that these patients shall have rest that they dose them with "considerable doses" of such sedatives as phenobarbital (luminal) and codeine. To aid in securing "rest" it is customary practice to whip up the heart with caffeine metrazol, coramine, epinephrine (adrenalin) and, though generally frowned upon in acute endocarditis, some physicians still employ digitalis in this condition.

In rheumatic endocarditis we learn from the "authorities" that "drugs other than salicylates, etc., are usually of little value." But they do use the ice-bag, and hot applications to "keep the patient quiet." If these don't "quiet" him, opiates are resorted to. It will thus be seen that no real rest is permitted the patient.

The latest medical text-books (editions of the Fall of 1943) admit that removal of the tonsils is ineffective in preventing a recurrence of acute endocarditis. Indeed one authority tells us that very few physicians are willing to deny serious and even fatal flare-ups of rheumatic affections, including those of the heart, are "sometimes suspiciously associated with" removal of the tonsils. Some of the authorities, who, in 1927 were sure the tonsils should be removed in every case of rheumatic fever, by 1940 had reached the point where they were less sure of this.

Drugs also fail to remedy endocarditis. Medical authorities are agreed that "no form of treatment is successful," and that "we have no effective medication in the heart failure of acute endocarditis and had as well admit it."

Two vivisectors in Mt. Sinia Hospital (New York), using heart patients as guinea pigs in experiments with the sulfonamides, report that:

Of 200 *patients treated with the sulfonamides,* 94 *per cent died.*

Of 43 *treated with sulfonamides and heparin,* 88.5 *per cent died.*

Of 45 *treated with sulfonamides and fever therapy,* 75 to 84 *per cent (they should make up their minds which) died.*

They claimed to have a larger number of "recoveries" (they probably mean survivals) when they employed the typhoid vaccine to induce fever than when they employed *hyperthermia*, which is a highbrow term for heat.

We are informed by the "authorities," that the small and differing numbers of cases in these series make it impossible to derive any statistical conclusions from them. Personally, I think they are wrong. I think the high death rates in each series show, unmistakably, that neither of these methods of treatment has any value. Other vivisectors, trying out the combination of sulfonamides and heparin had a high percentage (8 out of 22) of cerebral hemorrhage. They "question the advisability" of further use of the method. Nonetheless all of these methods are now in use, and the latest medical text-books advise them.

"Truly a Pain in the Neck"

The above is part of the heading of an item in the *Sunday Pittsburgh Press* (Dec. 12, 1943). The rest of the heading says: MEDICAL JOURNAL EXPLODES TONSILLECTOMY CURE-ALL. For a sub-heading we have: "Wholesale Tonsil Operations, with Adenoids on Side, Attacked by Physicians' Publication." The news item itself, follows:

A large proportion of tonsil and adenoid operations are unnecessary, and they should be greatly reduced to ease the wartime pressure on doctors and hospitals, declares a frank editorial in the Pennsylvania Medical Journal.

Tonsillectomies, the editorial reveals, account for about one-third of all surgical operations and lead all other conditions in demand for hospital service.

There are cases in which a tonsil operation is warranted, the editorial explains. But —

"Since there is no acceptable evidence that the indiscriminate removal of tonsils benefits the patient with arthritis, nephritis, rheumatic fever and heart disease, or with diseases of the eye, and since the incidence of colds and pneumonia is not reduced by the operation, there would seem to be no need for its wholesale perpetuation."

Furthermore, the editorial asserts —

"Error should not be made in diagnosing the natural state of hyperthropy (enlargement) of the tonsils in childhood as evidence of 'infected

—111—

tonsils' simply because they are enlarged. They rarely become large enough to interfere seriously with breathing or eating, and it is rarely possible by inspection to state with certainty that the tonsils are 'infected.'

"It seems plain _____ that a large proportion of tonsil and adenoid operations now done are unnecessary, entail some risk, and give little or no return. Furthermore, a great reduction in the operation rate would be followed by no unsatisfactory result, and it may be by actual benefit. It would certainly go far in relieving the crowded hospitals."

The editorial concludes with a suggestion —

"One way to bring about the desired result is suggested by the experience of Denzer and Felshin, who established a 'pre-tonsillectomy clinic.' Of 217 children referred to their hospital for tonsillectomy and passed through this clinic, tonsillectomy was permitted after careful investigation in only 17 per cent."

Now that physicians, surgeons and hospitals are worked to capacity, they are willing to give up part of their racket. They have known for years that there was not the slightest justification for their wholesale butchering of the tonsils. But they were not willing to discontinue so profitable a crime. Only, now, that they can make plenty of money without it, are they willing to give up part of the racket.

That they are not willing to tell the truth, *that there is never a time or condition when removal of the tonsils is wise, beneficial or necessary,* and discontinue the criminal practice, is evidenced by the suggestion that the "pre-tonsillectomy clinic" with perhaps 17% of tonsils removed is good practice.

Running suspects through a "pre-tonsillectomy clinic" means money to the physicians, expense and worry to the parents, apprehension to the

children and serves no good of any kind. Removing the tonsils from 17% of those run
through the "bull pen" still represents a lot of
crime.

The *Pennsylvania Medical Journal* is twenty-
five years late with its alleged "exploding" of
the "tonsillectomy cure-all." It probably would
not have "exploded" the myth, even now, had
not war conditions made it necessary that something be done to lighten the load on the physicians left in civil life.

Readers of the *Review* have known all along
that removing tonsils to cure disease is only a
racket. Those who have read my book on tonsils and adenoids are fully informed about the
racket.

We would remind the *Pittsburgh Press* that
tonsil removal is much more than a mere "pain
in the neck" — that in addition to being a complete failure as a cure for arthritis, rheumatic
fever, etc., the operation has resulted in much
positive damage and in hundreds of deaths.

Peptic Ulcer —
Cause and Remedy

It is estimated that "one in ten" people of the United States has peptic ulcer—that at this time some 13,000,000 persons in this country either now have or have had such ulcers, while many who do not have them are building them. Indeed "stomach" ulcer is said to be the *number one* disease in America, outranking, overwhelmingly, such headliners as heart disease, tuberculosis, cancer, and Parran's boogey man, "syphilis."

I do not know how accurate the above statistics are. If we are to judge by past performances in the various medical campaigns, they are much too high. It is my judgement that a move is now under way to begin a nation-wide publicity campaign to frighten the people about "stomach" ulcers. The one thing that may prevent this campaign from assuming flood-like proportions is the admission that the medical profession knows "appallingly little" about the condition. If they were strictly honest they would admit that the little they do claim to know is very doubtful. For instance there seems to be some agreement among them that ulcers are due to "high pressure" living; yet they admit that it has no age barriers and is today increasing alarmingly among persons of all ages. One medical propagandist tells us of stomach ulcers that "once primarily the ailment of top-flight executives over 40, the condition is now found as readily among boys no older than the one who delivers your Saturday groceries."

If these facts be true, then, either the term "high pressure" living must be broadened to cover more territory than it has ever covered in the past, or else it must be admitted that the assumption that it is a "scourge resulting from 'high pressure' living" must be abandoned.

If it was formerly a "disease of middle life" and has now become a "disease of all ages" — of young and old alike — this must be due to the fact that the real cause of ulcers, once largely confined to older people, is now common in all ages of life and all classes of society, not merely in the top-flight executives.

Physicians admit they don't know the cause of ulcers. But they are sure they know what does not cause them. We learn from the above mentioned medical advertising man that smoking tobacco is "among the alleged causes of stomach ulceration" which "is said to be able by itself, to give rise to the condition," that is "bruited about by the heedless and ignorant." He names other "alleged causes" that are "bruited about by the heedless and ignorant." And then says "Practically any physician will tell you that not one of these, of itself, is a causative agent for ulceration of the stomach."

This statement, as it stands, cannot be allowed to go unchallenged. A causative agent may be one of several factors that collectively constitute cause. To say that tobacco using cannot be a factor in the production of gastric ulcer is equivalent to saying that its use has no deleterious influence upon health. This would be false. For tobacco not only impairs the general health, it also has a marked deleterious effect upon the stomach itself.

Among the other "alleged causes" mentioned by the advertising man are "eating starchy and rich foods, eating fried foods, eating only highly seasoned foods, an indiscriminate diet, an inadequate consumption of food, too much pork, drinking liquor, excitement and worry, 'nervous' stomach, indigestion, chronic constipation, and frequent gas attacks."

Here we see an indiscriminate jumbling together of injurious practices and some of the earlier effects of these practices. We are assured that "not one of these, of itself, is a causative agent for ulceration of the stomach." We are of the opinion that the writer was trying to say that not one of these, of itself, is the cause of ul-ation of the stomach. We could agree with that. But if he intends to deny that any one of these habits of eating, drinking, smoking and wor-rying does not and cannot contribute to the production of gastric ulcer, we do not agree.

Indigestion, "nervous" stomach, chronic con-stipation, and frequent gas "attacks" are effects — not causes. They are links in a chain of patho-logical developments that may end in ulcer or in appoplexy. There is no better beginning out of which to evolve a peptic ulcer than that of chronic indigestion — *gastritis*. But the indigestion is not cause. It is a step or stage in the patho-logical evolution.

Ulcer is an end-point in a process of patholog-ical evolution that had its beginning in infan-cy. The first cold of infancy represents an estab-lished toxemia that sticks with the individual throughout life.

The first digestive upset — gastritis — of infancy may pass away without leaving any marks. But after repeated "upsets" the catarrh — gastritis — tends to become chronic. Then, the more such stomachs are abused by alcohol, tobacco, spices, imprudent eating, worry, etc., the worse the catarrhal inflammation becomes until, finally, ulceration occurs.

Ulceration is one of many possible endings of chronic toxemia. Toxemia results from inhibition of secretion — elimination — by enervation. Enervation is the sum of the effects of all our behaviour that collectively expends nerve energy in excess. Overeating does not cause gastric ulcer; it causes enervation. Tobacco does not cause gastric ulcer; it causes enervation. Alcohol does not cause gastric ulcer; it causes enervation. Worry does not cause gastric ulcer; it causes enervation. Enervation does not cause gastric ulcer; it causes toxemia. Toxemia is the cause of gastric ulcer.

Organs that are congenitally weaker, or that are most stressed by habit, environment or toxemic crises succumb to toxemia first. Overeating stresses the stomach. So do alcohol, tobacco, spices, imprudent eating and many other factors. Thus, these factors may help in two ways to produce ulcer. But so can a thousand factors help to produce ulcer.

"Top-flight executives" are notorious for their heavy smoking, drinking, hurried eating of wrong food, and bad tempers. These things can help to produce gastric ulcer in such men. What has the spread of smoking, drinking, coffee using, hot dog eating, and heavy condiment using among the young to do with the increasing incidence of gastric ulcer among this class of citizens? If formerly the young indulged in these things so little that they did not build ulcer before middle life; are they now indulging so much that they are building ulcer much earlier?

It is a fact that thousands of young men have been rejected for military service because either they've had ulcers, do have ulcers or are building ulcers. Many others have been discharged from the military and naval forces after developing ulcers while in service. As the medical profession does not know what to do for the condition, no time is wasted on these cases.

Our propagandist tells us that "nearly every doctor (he means physician) has his own pet theory as to the cause of stomach ulcers. There is not as yet any general acceptance of any of these as definitely specific." There is no such thing as a specific cause for any so-called "disease." The simplest "disease" is the complex effect of many correlated factors. The cause of gastric ulcer will forever elude the men of medicine so long as they continue to search for a "definitely specific" cause.

We learn that there is some general agreement about two causes of ulcers. For instance: "*since there are many cases where several members of a family are affected with the disease a hereditary factor seems to be involved in it.*"

Do we conclude that a hereditary factor is involved in the cause of frostbite because we find many cases where several members of a family are afflicted with it? "Moreover, a broad view accepted by most physicians, is that every sufferer from this ailment is from birth possessed of a stomach peculiarly susceptible to the condition and growth of ulcers." This "broad view" is "accepted" because of their ignorance of the real cause. Next: "The medical profession is nearly in agreement now that in many cases, stomach ulcers are, in a large measure, caused by mental disturbances — worry, tension, nervousness, and a generally unbalanced emotional state." If they are so agreed, is it not about time they ceased treating the condition with drugs and knives?

Our propagandist says: "Physicians do know the various types of stomach ulcers and how to treat and heal them, but the medical profession does not know what the precise causative agents responsible for the condition are nor how to eradicate it permanently in an individual."

Healing is a vital process. No physician can heal an ulcer any more than he can heal a wound or a broken bone. To say that a physician can heal an ulcer is to display a type of ignorance that belongs to the Dark Ages. To assume that a condition can be healed without removing its cause is to display a faith in the magic of the voodoo that is unworthy of children. Such statements are misleading and serve to emphasize the fact that men should not attempt to write upon subjects about which they are ignorant.

He does add: "If a doctor tells you he can *cure* an ulcer in your stomach, you'd better hunt up another M.D. He is not being honest. *There is no permanent cure for stomach ulcers.* While it is possible to heal a stomach thus infected there always remains latent the possibility that, regardless how strict a dietary care is exercised, the condition may recur at any time."

Although not originally having the same meaning, the words *heal* and *cure* are now used synonymously. Our hack says the physician can heal the ulcer but he cannot cure it. It would be interesting to know just what he means. He then says that, while the physician can heal the ulcer, there is no permanent cure for stomach ulcers. Then he hints that the ulcer may be due to an infection — bacterial invasion — that may remain latent in the "cured" cases and go on a rampage again when least expected, despite all precautions.

There is no physician who can cure any so-called disease. The man who promises to cure anybody of any so-called disease is either a fool or a knave; that man who believes him is a fool. Curing disease is a voodoo trick that belongs to the unenlightened past. Well informed people no longer believe in such magic.

Nature heals when cause is removed. Healing work is always going on. Its success depends on removing cause. Its permanence depends on permanent removal of cause. Permanent freedom from stomach ulcers depends on permanent reform in the whole mode of life. "Strict dietary care" (which is usually an abomination) does not constitute a reformed mode of life. This alone is not enough to guard against the recurrence of ulcers. Only by not again building toxemia can we be sure of not again building ulcer. *First class habits alone can guarantee us against rebuilding toxemia.*

The drunkard who has sobered up can stay sober if he refrains from drinking. But there is no permanent soberness for the man who, once sober, returns to drink. It is nonsense to discuss *permanent cure* when they know nothing of cause.

Returning to our hack, he says: "A physician can heal an external ulcer with comparative ease; but treating an ulcer deep within the body is a very complex matter. *And rare, indeed, are those instances of ulcers healing without medical treatment.*"

This writer is doing a difficult and delicate job of tight rope walking. He is both trying to tell us that physicians know nothing about the cause of ulcers and cannot *cure* them and that at the same time they can *cure* them and that it is almost impossible to get well without medical treatment. He has been assigned a difficult task, one that only a de Kruif can do with *finnesse,* and he is having difficulty staying on his tight rope.

He is obviously ignorant of the first thing about the process of healing. If this were not so he could not say that "a physician can heal an external ulcer with comparative ease." He would know that a physician cannot heal anything. Also, if he would look around him and see the many cases of external ulcer that have persisted for years "in spite" of the "healing" ministrations of physicians, he would develop a wholesome doubt of the ease with which physicians do the things they have told him they do.

If his last statement had been: *rare, indeed, are those instances of ulcers healing with medical treatment*, he would have told the real truth. The rule is "operate after the ulcer has been cured nine times." This kind of "healing" is not true healing and should not deceive anyone. Medical treatment cannot heal an ulcer, nor can it facilitate healing for the reason that it does not remove the cause of the ulcer. Medical men cannot remove the cause of ulcers for the reason that they do not know the cause. Their treatment is not intended to remove cause. They do not regard cause when they prescribe their doses.

So long as this is so, there is no sense in the statement he quotes from a "surgeon at the famed Mayo clinic", that "people must be taught that while stomach ulcers in a pair of individuals might be identical the methods of treatment will vary to meet the physical condition of each and their temperaments." This is bunk of the worst type. This business of "treating" patients differently according to their "physical condition" or their "temperaments," instead of removing the causes of their suffering, is also a hang-over from the past.

The surgeon gets rid of the above bit of malodorous gas after saying that there are people "who know their stomachs are ulcerated, yet seek to administer to themselves with remedies which proved effective in the case of a friend." All this mystery about "physical condition" and "temperaments", which he seeks to throw around the subject, seems to be designed to frighten sufferers into being treated by physicians, who confess they don't know the cause of the ulceration and cannot *cure* the ulcer. "We don't know anything about it, but let us treat you anyway."

Peptic ulcers are said to develop in the following locations in about the following percentages: in the duodenum, 90%; in the stomach and esophagus, 10%. They are said to be "of two broad types — benign and malignant." The malignant type is cancer, and is only another stage in the pathological evolution discussed above. Duoudenal ulcers are said to almost never become cancerous; gastric (stomach) ulcers are most likely to do so. The larger the ulcer the more likely it is to become cancerous, because there is more pathology and more cause of pathology.

Benign ulcers, like benign tumors, are pathologies and there is nothing benign about them. Benign ulcers, like benign tumors, may become malignant. The pathological evolution is always in that direction. We are informed that "Only an X-ray examination can determine whether an ulcer is benign or cancerous." This statement is misleading in that it implies that X-ray examinations are dependable.

Our hack tells us that the attitude of the medical profession is that "too much cannot be said and written about stomach ulcers; once the public is educated as to the *facts* about them our task is simplified. So ignorant are many sufferers of this condition and its seriousness that we must painstakingly explain the ailment as simply as one tells a child how and why the earth is round." He quotes this from some unidentified source. He, himself says: "Once an enlightened public learns to regard the disease as really serious, and to beware of its symptoms, it will be possible to cut drastically the high rate of its incidence nationally."

The incidence of ulcers can be reduced only by preventing them. Ulcer can be avoided only when its cause is known. A campaign to start people worrying about peptic ulcer and to get them to, in some mysterious way, "beware of its symptoms" will not enable anybody to avoid the cause of ulcers.

It is true the public is ignorant; but so is the profession that proposes to teach the people the "facts." How can the blind avoid falling into the ditch if the blind lead them?

Ulcers heal when toxemia is eliminated. Rest — mental, physical and physiological — and correction of all enervating habits and influences will allow the body to repair its damages and restore its health. There will be no recurrence of the ulcer if the restored individual does not return to an enervating mode of living.

Ulcerative Colitis

Itis is a little Greek word now used as a suffix to denote inflammation. When added to the name of an organ or part of the body it indicates inflammation of that organ or part. Thus inflammation of the stomach (gaster) is *gastritis*, inflamation of a joint (anthron) is called *arthritis*.

As the tendency of medical nosologists (nosos—disease, nosology, the science of disease and disease classification) is to create as many names as possible, the *itis* familiy has grown until the number of itises is very great.

To reiterate, "itis," when added to the name of an organ indicates inflammation of that organ. This is so simple a child may understand it; but when the medical classifiers get through defining all the numerous *itises*, and conferring upon each a personality all its own, the number of distinct diseases runs into the thousands and continues to grow in number.

It is as difficult for the layman as for the physician to comprehend the simple fact that inflammation (itis) covers the subject, wherever its location, and that the many itises do not represent as many different diseases. All seem to be unable to grasp the fact that inflammation in one organ is the same as inflammation in any other organ.

Colitis (colon, and itis) is inflammation of the colon. It is a catarrhal condition. We commonly hear it called mucus colitis because of the great amount of mucus excreted.

Rhinitis (rhino, nose and itis) is inflammation of the nose. It is a catarrhal condition and is also characterized by the secretion and discharge of much mucus. It is commonly called catarrh of the nose.

Is it difficult to understand that these two conditions (these two "diseases") merely represent the same condition in two locations — that instead of rhinitis and colitis being two "diseases", they are the same "disease" in two different organs? Is the simple fact of the *unity of disease* too complex for average understanding? Must we be forever misled by the confusing nomenclature of the schools of physic?

Colitis is simply catarrh of the colon; metritis is catarrh of the womb; cystitis is catarrh of the bladder; gastritis is catarrh of the stomach; rhinitis is catarrh of the nose; sinusitis is catarrh of the sinuses. Is this too simple for ordinary minds to grasp? Must the subject be made very complex before we can be duly impressed?

Inflammation in all these various locations is due to the same thing. Is it difficult to understand that a bee sting on the big toe of the left foot will cause inflammation and that a bee sting on the little finger of the right hand will cause inflammation? Different locations do not call for different causes of inflammation.

Toxemia is the cause of colitis as it is of rhinitis, gastritis, metritis, cystitis, phrenitis, arthritis, etc. What is toxemia? It is a blood and flesh condition in which the body is surcharged with metabolic waste — *metabolites*. It is a system poisoning (in-toxi-cation) resulting from autogenerated poisons.

When sensuality and emotionalism have brought on enervation, secretions and excretions are checked and the body becomes surcharged with the toxic waste products of the activities of life. Toxemia is a by-product of metabolism— is auto-generated and constant.

The enervation that checks elimination can come from any enervating cause or any combination of enervating causes. The particular combination of enervating factors that produces enervation and checked elimination in one case may be altogether different from the peculiar combination of enervating factors in another case. It does not matter what these causes are in any particular case so long as we understand that they all produce enervation, that enervation checks elimination, that checked elimination produces toxemia, that toxemia, when this is evolved, produces symptoms galore.

Elimination is a fundamental function of life —as fundamental as the processes of digestion and assimilation. Waste is carried out of the body as fast as the eliminating organs can excrete it. When enervation has reduced the functional efficiency of these organs and toxemia has been produced other and compensatory or vicarious channels of elimination must be established to rid the body of the accumulated toxins.

The cavities, canals, channels, ducts and sinuses are all lined with mucous membrane that secretes mucus. These membranes are excretory as well as secretory and when toxemia is established serve as emunctories through which surpluses and toxins are excreted.

This excretory process is called catarrhal inflammation. The classifiers and namers of "disease" bunch the symptoms and label them in keeping with the organ or location that acts as a fontannele.

Colitis is a process of compensatory elimination. The accumulated toxic waste is excreted by the membrane lining the colon or some part of it. It may be acute or chronic.

All chronic forms of catarrh begin as irritation, followed by inflammation, then ulceration. Instead of ulcerative colitis being a different "disease" than mucus colitis, it is merely an advanced condition or outgrowth of the latter. If the location of the ulceration favors stasis (blood stagnation), induration (hardening) and finally cancer (fungation) end life. Cancer, like ulceration, is an evolution out of chronic inflammation.

Cancer of the throat, cancer of the breast, cancer of the stomach, cancer of the liver, cancer of the colon, cancer of the womb (uterus), in fact, cancer in any part of the body evolves at a site of chronic inflammation. Over twenty per cent of ulcers of the stomach become malignant. Is it surprising to learn that ulcers of the colon or of the womb may also become cancer. Cancer may develop out of a prior hardening at a point of stasis without ulceration.

If we keep in mind the links in the pathological chain — enervation, toxemia, irritation, inflammation, ulceration, induration, fungation (cancer), we can, perhaps, understand how *cancer* has its beginnings many years before it finally appears. The "healing" professions wilfully or ignorantly flimflam their trusting patients in their treatment of all the initial and intermediate links of all pathological chains and, then, when the last link, malignancy, evolves, they label it cancer and write learned books of great size to explain their ignorance of the cause of cancer.

The fact is that cancer is a pathological potential of every cell in the body. Cancer is not a foreign organism feeding and growing parasitically off its host. It is a parasitic outgrowth of the body's own cells. To become cancerous these but require sufficient perversion of their metabolism, a thing that results from persistent excess of toxin saturated blood as seen in chronic inflammation in toxemic individuals.

Returning to ulcerative colitis, this simply means that ulceration of the mucous membrane of the colon has taken place. The inflammation has persisted and the parts have been taxed until ulceration developed.

If the cause of irritation, the toxemia, is corrected before ulceration occurs, no ulceration will ever take place. If the cause of irritation is corrected before cancer evolves, no cancer will put in its appearance. By this is not meant that chronically inflamed parts should be cut out. This surgical flimflamming of patients is inexcusable. X-ray and radium treatments both harden tisue; that is, produce the induration that is the beginning of malignancy in the pathological chain we have been discussing.

By correcting cause, we mean eliminating toxemia, restoring normal nerve energy and ordering the mode of living to conform with the laws of being. This is the "cure" for mucus colitis, and for ulcerative colitis as well as the prevention of cancer. Intelligent care will prevent the pathologic chain from ever reaching its malignant (cancerous) ending.

What is intelligent care? Remove cause is the only intelligent care. The usual palliative and suppressive care is unintelligent care — it is, in sober reality, abuse. It is care that helps to produce the malignant ending.

The body cures itself if the cause of autogeneration of disease is corrected. It should be understood that in all cases a point may be reached where organic change is great enough that the possibility of a return to normal no longer exists. Cause must be corrected before this point is reached if health is to be restored. After this point is reached all that can be expected from a removal of cause is a prolongation of life.

Bright's Disease

Acute and chronic nephritis (inflammation of the kidneys) receives the name, *Bright's disease* from Dr. John Bright, who first described it. Acute nephritis is largely confined to childhood and early youth; the chronic form is seen chiefly in middle life and beyond.

The symptoms of acute nephritis vary greatly. The inflammation may progress to a serious stage without the subject knowing he is sick. He may die suddenly; or, a few months later he may develop symptoms of chronic nephritis.

In many cases swelling of the ankles (dropsy), with the changes in the urine may be the only indication that something is wrong. The face is usually pale, and the eye-lids are puffy. There may or may not be pains in the back. Sometimes, though not always, there is headache. The sufferer may continue his regular duties not realizing he is very sick until, "suddenly," he becomes so ill he goes to bed and calls for a doctor.

In some cases, where the inflammation in the kidneys is not great, the symptoms are very severe. Chills, fever, nausea, vomiting, pains in the back and head, dizziness and weakness may be great in such cases. In other cases convulsions caused by uremia may be the first symptoms. In severe cases, dropsy, starting with the face and becoming general, and great anemia develop. Symptoms of uremia may develop at any stage of the "disease."

The urine is scanty, it may be wholly suppressed for a day or two. It is highly colored, cloudy, and of high specific gravity. Upon examination it is found to contain much blood, pus, casts from the kidneys, and large amounts of albumen. As improvement proceeds the amount of urine increases and the albumen, blood, pus and anemia and dropsy grow less.

The symptoms of chronic nephritis vary greatly in individual cases, and vary, even, in the same individual. Patients in advanced stages, with the kidneys largely destroyed, may go for extended periods without any symptoms at all. Even the small amount of functioning tissue that remains is capable of meeting the needs of life if not overburdened by a mode of living that swamps compensation.

The first indication of chronic nephritis may be a sudden uremic convulsion. The symptoms develop slowly and "insidiously." There is a progressive development of anemia with a gradual loss of strength. The walls of the arteries become thickened, the heart enlarges, digestive disturbances are frequent, there is headache, sleeplessness, dizziness and frequent uremia. Dropsy is often absent or it may appear late and be slight. It is often marked and chronic. In the late stages breathing becomes difficult. Inflammation of the retina, caused by the albumen, sometimes develops, producing dimness of sight.

There is much urine, of a pale color and of low specific gravity. It contains little albumen, few casts and occasionally some blood.

The amount of albumen in the urine varies so greatly that one can never judge by this how mild or severe the case is. An acute case may show so much albumen that when the urine is boiled it solidifies (coagulates). . The more chronic cases have less, and the most chronic cases have the least. The worst cases may show so little albumen that only an expert can find it, while, for months, all albumen may be absent. An acute case which recovers may have the maximal amount, while, a chronic case which dies may be present only a trace. Urinalysis may, therefore, be a most mis-leading index to the true condition of one who goes to the doctor for a periodic check-up.

Two forms of chronic Bright's disease are recognized — namely, *chronic parenchymatous nephritis*, in which the inflammation is largely or wholly in the functioning, or renal, cells of the kidneys, and, *chronic interstitial nephritis*, in which the supporting structures of the kidneys, the connective tissue, blood vessels, etc., are the structures inflamed. For practical purposes, whether for prevention, or for restoration of health, these distinctions are superfluous.

Medical authorities tell us that "acute Bright's disease gets well or kills within a few weeks. Chronic Bright's disease never gets well, but may persist with very fair health for ten or even twenty to thirty years." They point out that in most cases of acute Bright's disease the patient completely recovers, but that in some cases, the patient appears to get well, but the condition continues in the sub-acute or chronic form. It is our contention that these conditions result from mal-treatment and from a return to wrong living after apparent recovery.

The destroyed kidney cells cannot be replaced, though the remaining portions of the kidneys may enlarge and carry on their functions very efficiently. Cure depends on the amount of functioning tissue left. If sufficient functioning tissue remains to carry on the functions of life and the patient will learn to live within the capacity of the impaired kidneys, the progress of degeneration may be stayed and he may enjoy good health for many years to come.

Many destructive and degenerative changes occur in the kidneys and elsewhere in Bright's disease, but from a practical viewpoint, these changes concern us far less than do their causes. We are not so much interested in the nature of the degenerative changes as we are in the nature of the changes in the daily living habits of the patient, which are essential to the arrest of the degeneration. The really important question is what habits of living must be avoided in order to prevent these changes from developing in the first place and to prevent them from continuing, once they have begun.

Only rarely today does one possess typically healthy kidneys. Most people dying from other causes, have been, to a large extent, made less resistant to them by the all too common kidney degeneration. Few people realize what a tremendous tax the conventional mode of living places upon their kidneys.

Medical works, in stating the cause of Bright's disease, contain brilliant observations like the following: "Young persons and among adult males," "pregnancy." These are given as causes of both the acute and chronic forms, while we are sagely told that it "may occur without apparent cause." They also list "infectious diseases, especially scarlet fever," "acute tonsilitis, acute gastroenteritis, syphilis, and acute tuberculosis," as causes of the acute form, and, to these, they add, as causes of the chronic form, "malaria, septicemia, chronic suppuration or tuberculosis," "arteriosclerosis" and "passive congestion from heart disease."

A profession that can regard youth," "male sex," "pregnancy," and curative crises as causes of inflammation of the kidneys does not merit consideration and we consider them here only because the profession, being ancient and, therefore, honorable, has a large part of earth's inhabitants hypnotized into believing in them and their follies.

To the kidneys are carried most of the poisons that are produced in the body or that get into the body from without, for excretion. Upon them is thrown the greater part of the burden of keeping the bloodstream sweet and clean. Though naturally very resistant to toxins, they have their limitations and are finally broken down by the continued overwork and irritation they are called upon to bear.

All drugs, vaccines, serums, antitoxins, toxoids, gland extracts, etc., are renal irritants and Bright's disease is a frequent aftermath of serum inoculation. Tobacco, tea, coffee, chocolate, cocoa, alcoholic "drinks," soda fountain slops, turpentine, mercury, lead, arsenic, etc., are all destructive of kidney tissues and aid in producing pathology in these. Because the average person never checks on the amount and kinds of poisons he is deliberately introducing into his body, either as "medicines," or for "pleasure," and the frequency with which these are introduced, he does not adequately realize how much irritation he regularly subjects his kidneys to. Post mortem studies of the kidneys of those who died between the ages of fourteen and eighty years have shown that practically every kidney shows some structural damage.

Pus from teeth or tonsils is commonly held responsible for kidney "disease." The damage a little pus can do is as nothing compared to what the above poisons and the thousands of others given by physicians can do. The wholesale administration of vaccines, serums, and drugs is responsible for a large share of the cases of Bright's disease.

Sepsis habitually absorbed from the digestive tract is another common source of pathology in the kidneys. Abstemious livers do not develop this so-called disease. It is rather a *disease* of "high livers" and gluttons, those whose digestive tracts are constantly full of decomposing food-stuffs. Protein decomposition (putrefaction) is particularly prolific of virulent poisons that reach the kidneys for elimination.

Over-eating, frequent eating, eating without relish, eating wrong combinations of food, eating when digestion is impaired or suspended, eating when power to digest is absent — these forms of eating assure gastro-intestinal decomposition and septic infection of the body.

Eating candies, cakes, pies, jellies, jams, sugars, pastries, puddings, and the like, also favors fermentation and putrefaction and leads to intestinal autointoxication.

Perhaps few of the above causes would result in Bright's disease in a person of pure blood and full nerve force. But enervation and toxemia are so nearly universal that the resistance and functioning power of the kidneys are often very low. Enervation and toxemia should be considered basic or primary causes of Bright's disease with the above causes only auxiliary.

The fear and terror produced in the mind of the patient and members of his or her family by a diagnosis of Bright's disease are the results of the regular failure of the prevailing methods of treatment. These methods of treatment are all based on a study of the nature of the changes in the kidneys and not upon a study of the patient's habits of living, eating, and drinking and the relation of the kidneys to the nervous system, the digestive and circulatory organs and to body metabolism in general.

BRIGHT'S DISEASE

There is no chronic "disease" that responds so readily or so quickly to proper hygienic and dietetic care as chronic Bright's disease, while acute Bright's disease responds even quicker. When the "disease" is regarded as a degeneration resulting from a systemic toxemia and the sufferer is cared for with a view of eliminating all sources of toxemia, nephritis is not difficult to get rid of.

Acute Bright's disease is always a curable condition. Cases which have become wholly blind and in which there are delirium, convulsions, unconsciousness and much blood in the urine (symptoms of uremia) have recovered. There are always grounds for hope in the acute stages.

Rest in bed, with perfect quiet and no food but water until all acute symptoms are gone are the prime requisites. Feeding should not be resumed for at least forty-eight hours after all acute symptoms have subsided. No drugs of any kind for any purpose, should be allowed.

Feeding should begin with fruits for the first three to five days in very moderate quantities and the return to a normal diet should be made very gradually. Make haste slowly.

After the patient has gained considerable strength he may be permitted to get out of bed and gradually return to a normal mode of living, care being taken to prevent a return to the wrong living habits which produced the trouble.

Chronic cases require longer time for recovery than do acute cases. But persistence on the right road will result in recovery.

The first step should be to correct the whole mode of living. This is something medical men have never done. Their usual advice is "avoid excess of food and drink, alcohol and tobacco." No real dietary advice is given. What is an excess of tobacco? Of alcohol? How little is not an excess? Of what value is such advice?

What is the value of telling patients to avoid excesses of food and sending them home to eat white bread, cakes, pies, pastries, jellies, jams, denatured cereals, tea, coffee, fried foods, etc. What is the value of the customary advice to use salt sparingly? Salt causes kidney degeneration. It should not be used at all. Nor should we wait until the kidneys are greatly damaged before avoiding salt. Avoid it always and thus prevent the kidney deterioration.

What Are Tumors?

I despair of ever educating the medical profession. It is always a much easier task to educate uneducated people than to re-educate the miseducated. Irving S. Cutter, M. D., is an old man and there is certainly no hope thàt he can be educated.

It can hardly be said that he is so old that in his boyhood he knew the cave-man, but it may be correctly said that the cave-man is with us in "spirit," so that we are encumbered with a lot of intellectual lumber that he dumped on our mental shoulders.

In his syndicated article of July 21, Cutter discusses. *Brain Tumors* which, he assures us, are "no longer hopeless." His language about these growths is that of a *troglodite*. He says:

Tumors are ruthless. They do not regard any region of the body as sacred. They will barge into the most important structure, and the brain is no exception.

This language implies that tumors are some kind of foreign foe that invades the body from without and sets up housekeeping in the most inconvenient (inconvenient to the host) places. They do not respect the most "sacred" places of the body, these "ruthless" foes of ours.

Their's is a "sneak attack" like that of the Japs on Pearl Harbor. They are some unprovoked horror that pounce upon us from out of their secret hiding places.

The voodoo priests will never get away from their ancient belief that disease is an extraneous entity that attacks the body. Tumors are "ruthless" entities that "barge into the most important structures" and "do not regard any region of the body as sacred."

We could excuse such ignorant talk in a Hottentot or a Zulu, but a man who lives in America, has been educated in American schools and colleges, has been a professor in a medical college and who writes for the daily press of the country, can not be excused for this display of learned ignorance.

We know that Cutter is well aware of the fact that a tumor grows out of the patient's own tissues. Its cells and tissues are the patient's own cells and tissues. They do not come from without. They originate at the site of their growth. They are local mal-evolutions and are not "ruthless" foreign invaders.

A myoma is a tumor composed of muscle tissue; a lipoma is a tumor composed of fatty tissue; an osteoma is a tumor composed of bone tissue; a neuroma is a tumor composed of nerve tissue; an adenoma is a tumor composed of gland tissue. A tumor of the breast may actually secrete milk.

There is no reason why educated men should go on speaking of local pathological overgrowths of this kind as ruthless foreign entities that invade the body and manifest no regard for any region thereof. There is no reason why intelligence should be attributed to them, an intelligence such as is implied in the words: "they do not regard any region of the body as sacred."

As before stated, Cutter is too old to change either his conceptions or his expressions. To him "disease" will always be an attacking force. He will go on describing it in such terms. We are not sure about the younger members of the profession of voodoo. They have been brought up in these conceptions and trained in these expressions; but it may still be possible to make them see that both the conceptions and the expressions are false.

Cutter enumerates a few symptoms that may (and may not, for he says "there are several conditions which can imitate a tumor") indicate brain tumor, explains the necessity for the co-operation of the family physician, the neurologist, the X-ray specialist and the surgeon, and urges "early recognition and treatment of these brain-invaders."

What is the treatment? "Fortunately, because of our present knowledge of surgical procedures, many of these swellings can be removed in toto, with restoration of health."

Who ever heard of surgery restoring health? Cutter means only that when the tumor is removed, those symptoms due to its pressure on adjacent parts of the brain cease. This does not mean that health is restored. It may mean (but doesn't) that the patient's health is no worse than it was before the tumor evolved. It does not mean that the tumor is self-caused and that when it is removed its cause is removed also. It does not mean that there will be no recurrence.

He adds: "This means that growths within the cranium are not always malignant. Many may not resemble cancer. Some are injurious only because they take up room, cause pressure and interfere with nerve pathways."

There should be plenty of vacant space inside the cranium of the average voodoo priest so that a tumor would give rise to symptoms only after it had attained considerable size.

Tumors are divided into benign and malignant (cancer) and this tends to obscure the fact that the so-called benign tumors are also pathological.

Neither type of tumor ever develops in healthy tissue. We will make real advance when we learn to keep ourselves well so that we will not develop tumors. Advances in surgical knowledge, skill and technique represent advances in expediency. The fact that advances are being made in this direction indicates that no genuine effort is being made to advance in the other.

We are satisfied with an ever-increasing array of expedients when we should be striving for integrity. We are satisfied to have our tumors cut out after they have developed; we should be satisfied with nothing short of that degree of health that prevents the development of tumors.

Physicians, neurologists and surgeons are satisfied if they can remove the tumor without killing the patient (if the operation kills the patient he cannot come back later for the removal of a subsequent tumor). They are making no effort to teach the people how they may avoid the development of these neoplasms (new growths).

Like the dentists, they have made great progress in the creation of expedients. Our dentists are very skilled in drilling, plugging, pulling and straightening teeth and in making bridges and plates, but they have neglected to teach the people to preserve the teeth they have.

The people have asked for bread and the physicians, surgeons, dentists, etc., have given them stones. They have asked for knowledge and the professionals have given them a showy commercialism. The people ask for strength and the professionals have given them crutches. The people have asked for wisdom; the professionals have uttered goose-speech.

Curing Gallstones

The fallacy that drinking large quantities of olive oil, sometimes with orange juice, lemon juice or grapefruit juice, will dissolve gall stones and cause them to pass out will not down. Only recently a man came into the *Health School* and told me about having olive oil and grapefruit juice prescribed for him (by some naturopath) to dissolve his gallstones. A few days later a letter came from a man in St. Louis in which he says: "I have heard that olive oil and orange juice would eventually dissolve and pass them" —gallstones.

I shall never forget the first experience I had with this old piece of humbuggery. I had a woman under my care who was convinced she had gallstones. I was equally certain that she did not have said stones. She refused to go on with my directions until she could have an X-ray examination to determine who was right.

Visiting an X-ray specialist, she found him out and, upon leaving his office, she ran into an old friend of hers. She told the friend of her pains and why she had visited the X-ray man's office. The friend told her of a physician who could quickly rid her of her gallstones and she went immediately to this man. He assured her that she had gallstones and prescribed for her. This man accepted her self-made diagnosis and she, therefore, knew that he was a man who knew what he was doing. I have no doubt that he knew what he was doing, but she didn't.

A few days later the woman came to my office with enough "gallstones" to fill two gall bladders and explained that she had passed many more—she only brought part of them for me to see. Some of these stones were larger than English walnuts and stones of such size could no more pass through the bile-duct than a horse can fly.

The woman was very happy — not only because she was now free of her stones, but, also, because she had proven that she had been right and I had been wrong in our diagnoses of her condition.

Taking one of the "stones" between my thumb and finger I crushed it. It was very soft. I smelled of it. It smelled like soap. I asked the woman to smell of it. She did. I asked, "what does it smell like?"

She replied, "That's a gallstone. I passed it."

I then asked, "Doesn't it smell like soap?"

She said, "Yes, but its a gallstone."

When, next I said, "The doctor you went to gave you a lot of olive oil to take," she replied that he did. I then explained that the excess oil had been converted into soap in her intestine and she had merely passed little balls of soap.

She refused to believe me. She would not give up her belief that she had passed gallstones, even after it was demonstrated to her that she had passed soap. She had gallstones on her mind and she would not give up her illusion.

Oil is made up of fatty acids. In the intestine the great excess of oil she took was combined with alkalies and the result was soap. Calcium soap, sodium soap and magnesium soap are the most common forms of soap thus produced.

As the excess of oil also has a laxative effect, the victim of this form of charlatanry and humbuggery often receives temporary relief from abdominal distress. This relief convinces them, also, that their "stones" have passed.

The fact that giving large quantities of oil results in the production of soap is well known to all practitioners of all the so-called schools of healing. Any practitioner who resorts to this method of *dissolving* and removing *gallstones* is a down right faker. He is deceiving his patients and taking their money under false pretenses.

I will not deny that there may be rare instances where the practitioner is justified in resorting to this deception as a form of mental treatment, although I have never seen such a case. Cases may exist where the "gallstones" are so deeply embedded in the mind that a catharsis of this kind is the most effective way of getting them out of the mind.

If such cases exist, they must be very rare, and they do not justify the use of the method in all cases of real or fancied gallstones. As regularly carried out the practice is one of the worst forms of humbuggery. Practitioners who resort to it should be fully exposed.

Gallstones, kidney stones, liver stones, pancreas stones, etc., result from perversion of metabolism. The real cure is to restore normal metabolism. Normal metabolism will dissolve the stones. The tendency of an excess of oil is to further impair metabolism. Such treatment does no good, but may do considerable harm.

Diabetes

If the people could be made to realize how little is really known by each and all of the schools of so-called healing about the cause of disease, instead of imposing their confidence in the professionals and overwhelming them with their plaudits and praise, they would insist that the whole crowd of them go jump into the lake together.

Today there is a great hullaballoo about the science of prevention; yet, how can disease be prevented if its cause is unknown? The ever-increasing prevalence of cancer, gastric ulcer, diseases of the heart and arteries, diseases of the brain and nervous system, Bright's disease, diabetes, etc., an increase that is often greater among physicians than among the laity, should convince all thoughtful people that this prevention does not prevent.

The curing programs are no better than the prevention plans. We have a whole group of schools of so-called healing — drugging schools and drugless schools — that are forever engaged in a fruitless effort to correct discomfort and eradicate pathology brought on by health-destroying habits, by drugs, serums, vaccines, manipulations, electrocutions, bakings, freezings, and various other slight-of-hand measures, while completely ignoring the health-impairing mode of living.

The veriest swain can prescribe intelligently if he can be made to understand cause. Without a knowledge of cause the wisest of men guess and experiment and, more often than otherwise, fall back upon some voodoo trick that they hope will cure in spite of a mode of living that builds disease daily.

I am not optimistic about the future. Now, as in the past, understanding of truth is for the few. The many will cling, as always, to the "idols of the tribe." If we can judge by man's physician and doctor worship and his universal belief in cures — the senseless and non-senseless cure-alls that are advocated, practiced and accepted as scientific medicine — the day is yet very far off when man will realize that he makes and unmakes himself.

Let us briefly consider that complex of symptoms (of un-ease) that has received the name *diabetes milletus*. Its incidence is everywhere increasing and the death rate in this condition steadily rises. Why should these things be so? Do we grow weaker as we grow wiser, or, is our profession of increased wisdom a mere boast?

Diabetes is a particular type of impairment, mild or severe, of metabolism. The body's ability to assimilate and oxydize sugar (all carbohydrates enter the blood as sugar) is impaired. As a consequence of this impairment of the body's ability to utilize carbohydrates, sugar accumulates in the blood and is excreted in the urine. It is thus lost from the body without being used.

The condition is blamed upon the failure of certain structures in the pancreas (the islands of Langerhans) to secrete sufficient of the hormone known as insulin. But to rest the matter here is to fail to find the true cause of diabetes. Pancreatic insufficiency is an effect. It is but a link in a chain. The real cause is back of this effect.

A noted British medical authority, J. E. R. McDonagh, says that diabetes "is an external manifestation of a chronic intestinal intoxication in which, in the end stage, the island cells of Langerhans may suffer destruction. Ridding humanity of a chronic intestinal intoxication would prevent diabetes and render insulin superfluous." I would emphasize that part of his statement which says the destruction of the Islands of Langerhans belongs to the final stage of diabetes, not to its early stages. There is often no destruction found in the pancreas after death.

There seems to be fairly general agreement among medical authorities that diabetes is due to some form of toxemia, but they do not attempt to discover the source of the toxemia and remove it. It is true that some attention has been given to the removal of purely secondary sources of toxemia (so-called "foci of infection") but, as these are not primary, the results have not been satisfactory.

Even intestinal intoxication (due to indigestion) is secondary and cannot be removed or eradicated without first eliminating the primary (or endogenous) toxemia arising from inhibited excretion. This cannot be eliminated, nor can digestive secretions be restored to normal without first overcoming enervation — that is, normal nerve energy must be restored. This cannot be done without first correcting the causes of enervation and this is never done.

The office of worry, fear, anxiety and other emotional stresses in crippling carbohydrate metabolism and causing the appearance of sugar in the urine, where previously there was none and increasing the sugar in those cases where sugar has already appeared in the urine, is well known, but to date there seems to be little recognition of the fact that this is due to the enervating effect of these anxiety states. That these states produce diarrhea or constipation, indigestion, headache and other symptoms at the same time they cripple carbohydrate metabolism is well known, but there is also little practical use made of the knowledge that emotional over-irritation cripples function generally.

Constipation is "relieved" with a laxative, indigestion is "relieved" with sodium bicarbonate, headache is "relieved" with aspirin, and glycosuria (sugar in the urine) is "relieved" with insulin. The toxemic state that is inevitably produced by the *destructive emotions* is ignored, even unrecognized, and is allowed to grow greater. Indeed, the very means used to "relieve" the above symptoms increase enervation and the consequent toxemia.

No doubt excess eating of sugars and starches places a heavy burden upon the pancreas and hastens its collapse, but we should recognize that this is only one of many ways that the functions of the pancreas are impaired. Each and every cause of enervation aids in producing functional and organic impairment. Nor should we forget that indolence is an equivalent of overeating.

Dominated as it is by the laboratory outlook, the profession has been content to direct its efforts to patching up the pancreas, which is but one of the organs of the body that suffer impairment of function and structure as a result of toxemia. It is hardly correct to say they patch up the pancreas. Rather, they seek merely to supply substitutes for pancreatic function and there are reasons for believing that this crutch further impairs the pancreas.

J. E. R. McDonagh, from whom we have previously quoted, says: "Diabetes is a symptom, not a disease, and insulin • • • does no more than palliate this symptom. The drug throws no light upon the cause, it does not act in the manner described, and, had the cause been found and eradicated as it can be, there would have been no need to use it."

Dr. Bedow Bayly, M.R.C.S., L.R.C.P., of England, calls the use of insulin in diabetes a "misapplication of knowledge" and says the truth of this "is seen in the mounting death-rate in all those countries into which it (insulin) has been introduced." In the face of this mounting death-rate, insulin (in the various forms now employed) continues to be the chief reliance of the medical profession in diabetes. They give insulin and ignore all causes. Indeed, they often actually encourage patients to continue in the pursuit of the very causes of enervation that constitute the ultimate causes of diabetes.

Insulin, as stated above, is a mere crutch. It enables the body to utilize the carbohydrates in larger amounts but it does nothing to remove the cause of impaired carbohydrate metabolism and it does not restore the functioning power of those parts of the pancreas that secrete insulin. To restore health means that the patient's own pancreas will supply his insulin needs. To employ insulin from animals is to palliate the symptom and encourage the deluded patient to continue in the way of life that leads down to the grave.

Returning to Dr. Bayly, he points out that with the all-flesh diet used in treating diabetes prior to 1910, the progress of the disease was rapid, that the method of starch reduction employed a few years later greatly reduced the death rate and that fasting still further reduced it. Then he quotes R. M. Wilder, M.D., as saying: "Diet remains the cornerstone of satisfactory treatment."

It remain true, however, that dietary manipulations are not satisfactory. That some diets are much superior to others in this condition is not disputed. What I want to emphasize, however, is that removal of cause (all causitive factors) is the corner-stone of all satisfactory care. Manipulating the diet and neglecting all the causes of enervation may be made, in some instances, to prolong life to a slight extent, but it will never restore health.

Perhaps it will not be amiss to point out in passing that most of the dietary manipulation that is done is of little or no real value. Many of these "diets" contain, in addition to an abundance of wrongly combined denatured foods, such harmful non-food substances as coffee, tea, cocoa, chocolate, beer, gin, ale, wine or other alcoholic drink, or the so-called soft drinks. Tobacco is rarely proscribed and over-eating is commonly encouraged.

These "diets" usually cater to popular tastes, prejudices and habits and are rarely designed to conform with physiological requirements. Dr. Tilden rightly says that "when the people are not sick, and are not out with a doctor's search warrant looking for a cure, they are sprinting like hell looking for sickness, and, as disease is a form of trouble, it is easily found." I would only add that their "doctors" are commonly seen in the vanguard of the sprinters, aiding in the search for disease.

Most of these "diets" revolve around a reduction or elimination of carbohydrates, particularly of sugars, and fail to provide adequately for the nutritive needs of the body. It is not unusual for them to result in increased troubles.

Fasting is an excellent and rapid means of ridding the blood of its load of sugar and it will enable the insulin user to abruptly discontinue the use of this drug, but fasting will not cure diabetes.

Fasting is an effective way of emptying the digestive tract of it load of putresence, thus ending intestinal intoxication. It also permits the elimination of toxemia. But this does not cure diabetes.

If rest is added to fasting, nerve energy will be regained and normal secretion and excretion restored. But this does not cure diabetes.

After these things have been done, diabetes will persist if the mode of living is unchanged. Recovery can only come when cause is corrected and cause is a wrong mode of life. Coffee and tobacco and other stimulants help cause it. Emotional over irritation and wrong diet help cause it. Sexual excesses and indolence help cause it. All causes must be removed. This done, the patient will evolve into good health.

Varicose Veins

"Medicine" has three favorite methods of treating varicose veins, not one of which seeks to remove the cause of varicosity; not one of which is designed to restore strength and tone to the walls of the veins. Two of these methods destroy the veins; the other is designed to support the veins and, in doing so, makes them weaker.

Surgical removal of the veins is one of the methods of destroying them. This methods is used very often. It is a confession of helplessness in the face of a comparatively simple abnormal condition.

Equally destructive and equally a confession of ignorance is the practce of coagulating the blood in the veins and rendering them unable to function. Sodium morrhuate is the preferred substance to inject into the varicosed veins to cause the blood to clot.

This injection method of treatment destroys the vein as effectually as does its surgical removal. Instead of restoring the vein to health and enabling it to function normally once again, these methods render it forever impossible that it shall ever function again. These methods are in line with traditional medical practices, all of which are destructive and all of which ignore causes.

When a vein is destroyed by either of these methods the other veins of the legs, especially the deep veins within the muscles, must carry the blood formerly carried by the destroyed vein. They must carry this blood in addition to their regular load. This puts an added burden upon veins that are probably also weakened by the same causes that had weakened the superficial veins.

The injection technique, itself, is comparatively simple, though not without danger to the patient, not the least of which is that of the escape of a blood clot into the general circulation to turn up at some place where it may produce much harm.

Considerable skill is claimed to be necessary to enable the physician to determine which cases are likely to prove "successful" when the injection is employed. Some varicose veins are said to be "unfavorable" for this method of destruction. In these cases surgical removal is usually advised.

The method of supporting and further weakening the veins is that of wearing elastic bandages. Some of these elastic supports are stockings. Others are cuffs but a few inches in length. Others are wrapped on like the wrap-on leggins we wore in the Army when we made the world safe for hypocracy the first time. I know a man who has been wearing these wrap-around supports for varicose veins for twenty years and his veins are worse than ever.

Regardless of which of these makeshift affairs is employed, they are intended only as supports and, while they are said to provide "complete safety", they do not remedy the condition. On the contrary, like all artificial supports, they further weaken the parts they support. In general they interfere with circulation in the parts on which they are worn.

A short tme ago, I saw a young pregnant woman who was wearing a short skirt. Her legs were wrapped from ankles to knees with wrap-on supports to palliate her varicose veins. It was a revoltingly ugly sight, but the young woman seemed to be unconcerned about the fact that she was advertising to all who had eyes to see and minds to understand, that she was slowly degenerating and doing nothing about it. She had placed herself in the hands of a physician and he knew not what to do to remedy her troubles

Varicose veins are frequently followed by wasting of the skin and underlyng tissues with the subsequent development of ulcers — varicose ulcers, as these are called. These are chronic and, under "regular"care, persist for years, often healing over and breaking open again repeatedly.

. Their failure to heal permanently is due to the fact that the causes that have produced them are never removed. The antecedent varicosities are not corrected, because their causes are not removed. Local treatments of the ulcers, both drug and surgical treatment, fail, because these do not remove the cause.

What are the causes of varicose veins? So-called "scientific medicine" (it is neither scientific nor medicine) does not know. It lists as causes such things as the following: the upright position, pregnancy in women, occupation, standing erect for long periods, lifting heavy burdens, heredity, phlebitis, tight garters and aging.

All but three of these alleged causes are normal, natural conditions and actions and the other three are "diseases". Three of these are effects, not causes. Varicose veins may be part of the aging process; the weakening of the walls of the veins may be caused by the cause of the phlebitis, it is not caused by the inflammation that receives this name.

That pregnancy is not the cause of varicose veins is shown by the thousands of women who go through several pregnancies without the slightest varicosity developing. That pregnancy plus the wrong eating and wrong care of this period may constitute the "last straw" in those women whose veins are already near the "breaking" point, we will not deny.

That standing erect for long hours causes varicose veins is a superstition that West Point Cadets should be told about. It is not standing erect or the upright position that causes varicose veins. Position can have an influence in this direction only after the veins are greatly weakened and are no longer able to carry their normal load.

Normally, all veins are capable of carrying much more blood than the ordinary activities of life require. They fail in their function and their walls begin to bulge only after they have been weakened and their functioning power is greatly weakened. When they have lost strength, tone and elasticity and their valves have been weakened they become varicosed, not before.

Heredity as a cause of disease is a myth. Heredity causes nothing. It is simply the transmission from one generation to the next of characters resident in the germ plasm. The average physician has not outgrown the pre-Mendellian ideas of heredity.

Inherited weaknesses constitute tendencies, not causes; but even these weaknesses have causes that are independent of heredity. It is doubtful that a tendency to varicose veins is ever inherited. It is most likely that any such tendency is due to faulty nutrition and lack of exercise, sunshine, etc., during the larval and later development stages.

The big cause of varicose veins, the cause without which they will never develop, is the gradual deterioration of the whole body as a result of wrong living. Enervation and toxemia account for varicose veins and these are caused by overeating, excessive fluid intake, overstimulation, and all other enervating causes.

Vigorous activity of the legs, as in brisk walking, running, jumping playing tennis, weight lifting, swimming, etc., build sound strong tissues in the legs and in the veins of the legs. Standing or sitting for long hours, without any physical activity, allows these same tissues to deteriorate. Daily exercise of the whole body, but especially of the legs will prevent this deterioration in those whose occupation calls for long hours of sitting and standing.

If pregnant women will eat less — if they will cease "eating for two" (six) — and will exercise more, they will not develop varicose veins. I have never seen the slightest evidence of developing varicosities in a single woman that I have guided through pregnancy. The real cause of varicose veins in pregnant women lies in their mode of life.

If we know the cause of varicose veins, we can remove it and watch the veins gradually become normal. A young lady (aged twenty) consulted me a few years ago who had rather marked varicosities on one leg. In addition to the changes made in her mode of living, I had her to run each morning for a distance commensurate with her strength. In one month her veins were normal.

To correct varicose veins, first correct all causes of enervation, then rest for recuperation of nerve energy; take a physiological rest and sunshine to build positive health.

"Relief" from Asthma

A man writes me that he has eight or nine "asthma spells" every day and that for the past three years he has been taking "injections of morphine" for relief. How "would you care for a person with asthma who takes so many injections," he asks.

The first step in caring for such a victim of criminal medical malpractice is to stop the injections. This man is a morphine addict, although he seems not to realize it. Some criminal started him on the road to addiction and he is now suffering more from morphine than with asthma.

He went to some professional product of a class A medical school who is licensed by a blind and ignorant state to poison and dope the sick—he went to this respectable and well-dressed criminal demanding "relief." The licensed dope peddler did not know the cause of asthma and how to remove that cause, so he gave him the desired "relief."

Today the poor victim of this ancient system of humbug and spectacular palliation is more in need of relief from his "relief" than he is in need of "relief" from his asthma. He is slowly killing himself with "relief". He is another sacrifice on the altar of the great therapeutic god — *Relief*.

He wanted "relief" and the dopester was determined to give him "relief" even if he had to kill him to do it. Just now the morphine is producing worse suffering than it "relieves." Morphine is popularly called a pain-killer (an anodyne); it is, in sober reality, a pain-producer (an *odyne*). It is a patient killer.

How can this man get well so long as he is enervating himself with frequent daily injections of morphine. Right now he is so profoundly enervated that there is little functioning power left in any of his organs.

He asks me to tell him how to free his body of toxemia. How? indeed! How can it be done in such a state of profound enervation while the enervation is being perpetuated and daily made worse by resort to fictional relief? Toxemia cannot be eliminated so long as the organs of elimination are depressed by morphine; so long as the nervous system is made and kept so weak by this dope that normal function is impossible.

We must depend on the organs of elimination to free the blood and lymph of its load of toxins. These are the only blood purifiers known. But they can't do their work well if they are only twenty or thirty per cent efficient. Where are they to derive functioning power from so long as the body is kept in a state of profound enervation?

We would not take such a man into the Health School unless he would abandon at once (abruptly) and completely, all use of morphine and any and every other poison he may be using with which to keep himself sick. We will not take dope addicts who are unwilling to abandon their dope.

The *Health School* is not a place where miracles are performed. We cannot suspend or set aside the laws of nature and make people well in spite of the continued operation of the cause of their illness. Every drug complicates the "disease" for which it is given.

Asthmatics are neurotics. Morphine produces worse neurosis. How can a neurotic recover from his neurosis so long as he is producing worse neurosis? At the *Health School* we have not found a way to accomplish this.

Asthmatics have poor digestion. Morphine cripples digestion. How can an asthmatic's crippled digestion be restored while it is being daily crippled with morphine? We don't know any form of magic, ancient or modern, white or black, by which this can be done.

Either all impairing causes are removed from the life of the sufferer or he continues to produce impairment and, so long as he is being constantly impaired, he can never be fully repaired.

The primary basic cause of asthma is toxemia. Toxemia is caused by many causes. The treatment this man is getting also causes toxemia. His "relief" perpetuates and intensifies his suffering. He can never get well until he abandons all enervating palliatives.

This victim of medical crimes wants to come to the *Health School* after he gets strong enough to travel. How is he to grow stronger on a program that daily makes him weaker? Morphine will not make him stronger. The longer his addiction is continued the weaker will be become. The more he is "relieved," the greater will grow his (apparent) need for "relief". "Relief" will kill him long before it makes him strong enough to travel from Pennsylvania to Texas.

A man so profoundly enervated and heavily toxemic as is this man, needs a prolonged period of mental, sensory, physical and physiological rest. Only by taking such rest can his nerve energy be restored and toxemia be eliminated. Only after the blood is pure and nerve energy is normal can he hope to build up by the use of proper food, exercise and sunshine.

Warts — Verruca

Warts are of several kinds, but the distinctions are unimportant. There are small, flat warts that develop principally on the face and back of the hands, chiefly of children, known as "juvenile warts," there are larger excrescences seen chiefly on the backs of the hands and wrists and sometimes on other parts of the body, known as *verruca vulgaris;* the *plantar wart* of the soles of the feet, the *filiform,* or narrow-based type of wart, developing principally on the face and scalp. Warts develop most often in children, but they may develop for the first time after adulthood is reached.

They are outgrowths of the papillae of the corium of the skin and the overlaying layers of the epidermis. A vascular (blood vessel) loop is found in the center of each wart.

Little is known about their cause. In medical circles they are said to be contagious and auto-inoculable. Both of these notions smack too much of the crude notions of past centuries to merit serious consideration.

The latest standard medical works say that "it is now believed that warts are caused by a filterable virus." After many years of intensive farming of the germ theory and getting nowhere with it, the voodoo crowd is now engaged in an equally intensive farming of the "filtrable virus" theory of etiology. We intend to discuss this absurd theory in a later article. At this point it is enough to say that the filtrable virus theory of the cause of warts is merely a belief. It has been a belief for a long time as reference to a

standard work on skin diseases published in
1921 shows. After the passage of 23 years it
is still only a belief.

My own theory of their cause is that they represent a perversion of nutrition, perhaps, often
as a result of local irritation. I see them frequently disappear spontaneously when the nutrition of the subject is corrected. They do not so
disappear in all cases.

As pointed out above, warts represent an elon-
gation of the papillae of the skin. They seem
to arise as a result of irritation, either from within
or from without.

British sheep growers noticed that their lambs
often developed a crop of warts on the mouth
and nose and on the tender part of the feet above
the coronet. Study showed that they had turned
their lambs into fields of clover in which stubble
from the previous crop of wheat remained. The
short, stiff, hard ends of the wheat straws irritated the above named parts and warts developed. When the lambs were removed from the
stubble the warts disappeared.

Those soft, hairless pads on the feet of the
carnivorous mammals, which permit them to walk
so noiselessly, are made up of closely packed,
enlarged papillae. When these animals are confined to cages and not kept scrupulously clean,
the combined effect of dirt and limited use,
often induces a growth of warts. In some of these
animals the whole pad will be so covered with
these elongated papillae, or warts, that they
give the appearance of the pad on the planter
side of the toe of the ostrich.

Small warts grow on the hands of children
when not kept clean. Grubbing about in dirt
and muddy, stagnant pools incidental to farm-
yards, will produce warts on the noses of lambs.
Similar digging around in the dirt, if not followed

by cleansing, is no doubt often responsible for warts on feet and hands of children.

It is very probable that many warts seen on the hands and faces of girls and women result from irritation produced by many cosmetic substances and that many warts seen on the faces of men are the results of the use of after-shaving lotions. Shaving creams that contain "skin conditioners" and other drugs may also be responsible. We are rapidly approaching the time when it will be impossible to buy shaving creams that do not contain drugs.

We see many warts in men and women where strict external cleanliness is regularly and habitually maintained. In such cases it may be concluded that internal toxic irritation is the cause of warts. I am strengthened in this view by the cases I have seen where the warts disappeared when the toxemia was eliminated and general nutrition normalized.

Medical methods are local treatments exclusively and designed only to destroy the growth. Fulguration (burning), usually with electricity, is the preferred method. X-ray and radium are also used, but these are frowned on by the best authorities because of their danger. Strong acids and injection of urea at the base of the wart are also used to destroy the growth. Some use suggestion and others treat the patient for "syphilis".

Our own plan is simple. External cleanliness is insisted upon. Thereafter every hygienic measure — fasting, improved diet, exercise, sunbaths, etc. — that favorably influences nutrition is employed. Where this alone fails to result in the disappearance of the warts we use the blue lens to concentrate the sun's rays upon the wart. One to a few such applications of the sun cause the wart to turn black and drop off leaving no scar.

Neurasthenia

One of the two great groups of troubles included under the term *psychoneurosis*, is *neurasthenia*. Neurasthenic individuals are crippled by fear and hesitancy; and are distressed with incapacitating aches and paralyzing dreads. It is now quite the fashion in medical circles to call these symptoms and weaknesses *imaginary*. They are referred to as neuroses and psychoses and commonly dismissed with the advice to forget them.

But the symptoms refuse to be forgotten. They are as real as any other type of symptom, rest upon a bed rock of cause, and stubbornly persist so long as cause is untouched and uncorrected.

Among the most prominent symptoms of neurasthenia are chronic tiredness or lack of strength and endurance, irritability, moodiness, depression, inability to concentrate, except on the work of introspection and critical analysis of symptoms, exaggerated pessimism, fear, worry, restlessness, headache, vertigo, visual disturbances, palpitation of the heart, cold hands and feet, hot flashes, insomnia, unpleasant dreams, etc.

Females often manifest a sense of social inferiority and a fear of mental unbalance. There is often irritation of the ovaries and painful menstruation. Males may present a fear of impotency (or be impotent) and there may be a genito-urinary obsession of some type. In both sexes there is likely to be constipation, often of the spastic type, and sometimes colitis. Frequent urination is often seen.

The symptoms are those of a profound enervation plus the resulting toxemia. Neurasthenia is also known as *nervous exhaustion* and *nervous prostration*. It is sometimes called the *American disease*. The many and varied symptoms grouped under this heading are due to the extravagant dissipation of energy in many useless ways and to the consequent self-poisoning. Energy is wasted to such a degree that the various functions of the body do not receive a full measure of nervous impulse. The result: digestive secretions, metabolism and all functional activities are impaired and a vicious circle of physical and emotional reactions becomes established from which these patients only rarely escape.

These patients make their own lives miserable and are a sore trial to their families, friends and physicians. The average physician contents himself with giving these patients "relief" from discomforts by the drug route and this serves only to increase the nervous exhaustion and the resulting discomforts.

The theory of enervation and toxemia in its entirety covers neurasthenia as it does that of all other so-called disease. It may seem preposterous to say that there is a simple beginning for every so-called disease and that this beginning, or cause, is identical in measles and in scarlet fever, that it is the same in a simple cold as in arteriosclerosis, but we affirm that this is so.

A cold is an acute catarrhal inflammation having its origin from within, even though the "exciting cause", which is usually some sudden enervating influence, may come or appear to come, from the outside. Arterial hardening is a late development resulting from stored-up wastes of exactly the same character. They have been accumulating for years, but they started in the same way as did those occasioning a cold. Auto-generated toxins and retained metabolic waste account for all of our so-called diseases. Is this more illogical than the assumption that measles, scarlet fever, smallpox (diseases for which no bacterial cause is known) are due to germs alone?

It is well known to medical men that the functions of an internal organ may be disturbed by toxic substances coming in contact with the peripheral portion of its nerve supply. It is also known that many drugs affect the vegetative nerves in this manner. Some of them have expressed the thought that when the various toxic processes that develop within the body are better understood, it will be found that these affect functional activities through the nerves just as drugs do.

And why not? Why will not irritation by autogenerated toxins produce as much functional disturbance as drug irritation? Certainly neurasthenics and others present the same kinds of functional impairments as drugs are known to produce. Poisoning, autogenerated, seems the most logical explanation.

It is well known that the body is never absolutely free of the waste products of metabolism. These are produced continuously so that, no matter how efficient the organs of elimination are, there are always waste products in the body. These become sources of trouble only when, due to impaired elimination, they have been allowed to accumulate in the body. It is our view that accumulated metabolic waste (toxemia) and absorbed poisons from septic intestines (autointoxication) supplies the toxic irritation that is the great factor in autonomic unrest. We know from experience that when toxemia is eliminated and its causes corrected, the symptoms of such unrest cease.

Headache, indigestion, abdominal pain, pylorospasm, spastic constipation, spasm of the rectal sphincter, heart palpitations, excessive intestinal peristalsis, hyperacidity, dilated pupils, increased blood pressure and other evidences of sympathetic nervous irritation cease when toxemia is eliminated.

I have repeatedly stressed many causes of enervation and toxemia. In this article I intend to stress the emotional causes. I do this, not because neurasthenia is due solely to emotional overirritation, but because the discussion of this trouble affords an excellent opportunity to stress the emotional factors of causation.

Man lives intensely and, it may be said, almost exclusively in his emotions. Where, then can we look for more constant and positive pathogenetic habits than in the emotional life of our patients? Here is a fruitful field, cultivation of which will yield as much as the nutritive field.

How frequently do our emotions influence, even absolutely dominate, our functions! Powerful reactions are produced by the major emotions, proportionate stirrings follow in the wake of the minor emotions. The physical responses to emotional processes are many, varied and complex. This is especially true of all those physiological functions controlled by the vegetative or autonomic nervous system. Emotions accelerate, suspend, or even, arrest function.

Functional impairments of emotional origin are all too common and the doctor or physician who fails to take into account the all-important factor of his patient's emotional habits, as well as his other personal habits, will be always working in the dark and will fail to lead his patients back to health.

An unpoised state of mind, or, rather, of emotions, saps one's energies and shortens life. This is not only true of those self-centered and grossly selfish individuals whose petty bickerings and disappointments make life miserable for all around them; but, it is also true of those larger, more noble, far seeing and philanthropic individuals whose larger disappointments arise out of the failure of truth to get a hearing or who are sickened by the gross inequalities and glaring injustices all around them.

The late Dr. Weger well said "one is either poised or poisoned." He emphasized that he meant this literally and not as a mere figure of speech. The waste of energy that results from a lack of poise produces enervation and, thereby, builds toxemia. Emotions interfere directly with the functions of the body and produce symptoms of their own which are aggravated by the resulting enervation and toxemia.

The cultivation of poise becomes, then, one of the great ends of life. The old philosophers, perhaps, builded better than they knew in this respect; our modern teachers have failed us precisely where we need them most. Our modern age is one of rush and excitement, of disappointment and frustration. Never was there more urgent need for the cultivation of poise; of emotional stability and equilibrium.

Well does Dr. Weger say: "The unpoised mind, coupled with a lively imagination, is often busy getting nothing from nowhere, or going from nowhere to no place, from void to vacancy, from uncertainty to inconsequence". No man is more conscious of the truth of this observation than the doctor who deals with impressionable and imaginative patients who exaggerate their symptoms, who are always seeking for new symptoms and fearful of tomorrow. They stand in their own way and prevent their own recovery. Time, patience, sympathetic understanding and tactful re-education of these patients are essential. Pills and powders do no good. It is not enough to tell them their symptoms are imaginary. Their symptoms are real; let there be no mistake about that.

"Modern medicine" built a gigantic system of spectacular palliation upon the false foundation supplied it by Pasteur and neglected the important branch of physiology that deals with man's endogeneous reactions upon his own body and its functions. Medical men derided Mesmer and Eddy and stuck to their pills and powders until forced, by loss of patronage, to give some reluctant attention to the *psychic* factors of man's life.

The pathogenetic influence of many emotional states, the healthful influence of many other emotional states were known long before the days of Pavlov, Cannon and Freud, but they were scarcely considered by the men of medicine. Beaumont long ago demonstrated the effects of emotional states upon digestion, but no one outside the ranks of the *Hygienists*, even yet, makes any practical application of this knowledge.

Do medical men, osteopaths, chiropractors, physio-therapists, naturopaths, the so-called mental therapists, etc., advise not eating when in mental and emotional distress? If so, I have not met with the advice and practice. Dr. Weger, who forsook the practice of medicine for the practice of *Hygiene,* says: "If emotional unrest of any kind interferes with the digestive, secretory, and other functions of the body, it is quite obvious that we must be poised or become poisoned".

If the major emotions produce grave digestive disturbances and the minor emotions give rise to lesser disturbances, the difference being only in degree, how can food be well and efficiently digested if eaten when one is fearful, worried, angry, fretful, irritated, apprehensive, grieved, enraged or full of self-pity? Poise means good digestion. Lack of poise means impaired digestion.

There is such a vast amount of evidence that mental conflicts and emotional disturbances upset normal physiological functions, both in children and in adults, and that where this upset persists, organic change may take place, that no man who contents himself with giving his patients arsenic or sulfa drugs or with "adjusting" their spines or giving them herbs or hot and cold baths and neglects emotional and other habits should be permitted to go on pretending to care. for the sick.

If causes are not corrected, recovery cannot take place. If the symptoms are of emotional origin, of what value is a pill or a bath? Of what value is a diet, even the best of diets, if emotions prevent its digestion and utilization? Failure must follow every neglect to find and correct and remove cause — any and all causes.

Dr. Weger puts it this way: "If patients persist in holding on to destructive emotions, thereby interfering daily with normal function, they will injure themselves much less by taking a restricted diet than if they gorge to repletion in the conventional way. Thus, we may conclude that unless a person can cure his mental waywardness, he must restrict himself as to food, for much food will kill more quickly in the presence of the same emotion".

Dr. Weger, in fact says of the neurasthenic that "fasting is his remedy and will be good for him in many ways". Unfortunately large numbers of the neurasthenic group insist on gorging themselves daily, even several times daily, in spite of the fact that they know they suffer every time they do it. Morbid *appetencies* and wayward emotions combine to create pain, discomfort and impaired function throughout their bodies.

NEURASTHENIA

In the care of **neurasthenic** subjects due consideration is rarely given to the existence of toxic saturation. The office of **toxic** irritation in producing the thousand and one neuroses and psychoses with which these subjects suffer is all too commonly overlooked. Psychological "treatment", important as this is in re-educating and reshaping the emotional life of the patient, is almost never enough to restore these cases to health. Toxin elimination is of basic **importance.**

In addition to emotional re-education and toxin elimination it is essential to restore full health by the employment of all the positive hygienic factors with which life is sustained and function carried on.

Influenza

Influenza is defined as a "contagious epidemic catarrhal fever with great prostration and varying symptoms and sequels: grippe, or La Grippe." After the utter failure of the efforts to transfer influenza from one person to another by the many means tried in 1918-19, it seems that the word "contagious" should be omitted from the definition.

Indeed, it is my conviction that the word "influenza" and the thought that there is such a disease should be forgotten. It seems to be a vogue rather than anything else. I have met but one person in all San Antonio this season who had a cold. All the others had "the flu." If they sneezed as many as three times during the day, they had "the flu." I frequently heard them say: "I am taking the flu."

Influenza epidemics are started by physicians and, once they get an epidemic started, both they and the public label every trouble that comes, "the flu." No more forceful example of this fact can be offered than the pandemic of 1918-19. At that time everything from a mild cold to sleeping sickness was diagnosed as influenza. Physicians were called to see patients in the early stages of their troubles and, without waiting for full developments, diagnosed everything "flu." Then, when a day or two later, they found they had pneumonia, or meningitis or sleeping sickness on their hands, they said these were complications of the "flu."

In France a lot of our boys died of "flu." At autopsy it was found they had died of typhoid fever. The physicians were not, of course, expect-

ed to find typhoid fever in well-immunized men.
"Flu" was in fashion, so their diagnoses conform-
ed to the fashion.

Thousands of "flare-ups" in cases of so-called
arrested tuberculosis, were diagnosed as "flu."
Influenza is a blanket term, which, like the terms
"syphilis," "rheumatism," "neurasthenia," and
"chronic appendicitis," is applied to a multitude
of symptom-complexes. It has no settled meaning
and should be dropped from our language.

We read that the "onset" of influenza begins
with fever, sometimes with a chill. The term,
"onset" is a hangover from the days when diseases were entities that "attack" us.

The symptoms are those of a severe cold. Indeed, we are told that "the difference between
influenza and an ordinary cold is the tendency
of the former to continue long after the time for
a hard cold to disappear." The "victim" complains of being very weak and in some cases
the weakness runs on for weeks and the catarrh,
which is always pronounced, hangs on continuously. In pronounced cases, the mucous membrane
is involved from the nose through the entire
bronchial tubes; the lungs often become engorg-
ed. Pneumonia and pleurisy often develop. Delirium and prostration are often present, in those
cases in which the bronchial tubes and lungs
are involved. The so-called nervous forms of influenza are characterized by headache, much
pain in the joints, and prostration. Other cases
"develop in a manner similar to that of typhoid
fever." "Intestinal influenza" is marked by much
fever and by such "complications" as pericarditis, endocarditis, septicemia, peritonitis, etc.

Epidemics represent mass sickness. There is
much more than the usual amount of sickness
due to some added general prostrating influence,
such as war. There is an increase in all forms of
illness, but one of these is headlined. Colds are

more severe and last longer when the people are enervated and, as a consequence, more toxemic. They last longer and develop more complications when the patients receive more heroic treatment.

Major Austin of the British Army Medical Corps, tells us of his experiences with "influenza" in 1918. He says that "during the virulent influenza epidemic in Calcutta in the cold weather of 1918" twenty of his cases volunteered to try the fasting "cure." The fasts in these cases lasted four to six days. "No drugs were administered during the treatment other than a saline purge, which was taken daily during the fasting period." He tells us that "within eight to ten days these cases were all fit and strong enough to return to their work, and they had excellent appetites for even the plainest of meals."

His other cases did not fare so well. Of these, he says: "I was not so fortunate, however, with other cases of influenza which had text-book diet —milk, beef-tea, egg-flip, etc.—— from the beginning of the disease.

"Few of them escaped the text-book complications — gastritis, bronchitis, pleurisy, or pneumonia — while one got double pneumonia and died. Most of them were unfit for duty for two or three weeks, and some very much longer."

Physicians and patients rarely realize how much the treatment is responsible for increased and prolonged suffering and for death. Physicians are unaware of the fallacy contained in their advice to "eat plenty of good nourishing food to keep up your strength." Few of them realize the truth of the statement made by a leading physician during the last century that, "thousands are annually slaughtered in the quiet sick room."

Delirium, spasm, peritonitis, pneumonia, pleurisy, heart trouble, sleeping sickness, etc., are listed among the "complications" of "influenza." These develop in those who are fed and drugged. Complications are treatment-made. Physicians should feel very proud of their ability to build pathology; to make two diseases grow where only one grew before.

The different so-called catarrhal fevers — colds, influenza, etc. — are one and the same, differing only in degree. Enervation and toxemia complicated by much intestinal decomposition are the causes. The most enervated, hence the most toxemic, have the severest cases and in this class is also seen the highest mortality rate.

Those who live prudently will not develop "influenza." Sensualists and gluttons will suffer most. Feast days — Thanksgiving and Christmas — are followed by epidemics of acute disease. The lesson is obvious. Eat moderately and keep well.

Before the 1918-19 pandemic, the physicians of the world knew exactly what causes influenza. The causative germ had been discovered, described, labeled and pointed out to the physicians and bacteriologists. But when the pandemic developed, the microbe proved to be a very contrary fellow. He was present where he should have been absent, absent where he should have been present, and failed to produce the disease when given to volunteers in a variety of ways. Physicians and bacteriologists came to the conclusion that they had tagged the wrong microbe. After more futile search for the guilty microbe, they decided that influenza is due to a "virus," and there the matter has been allowed to rest. They are back where they started from some thousands of years ago — diseases are due to evil spirits.

The influenza-pneumonia pandemic of 1918-19 left a trail of death and devastation in its wake. More people died in six months than were killed in four years of war. In some localities the death rate was above sixty per cent. Medical treatment was responsible for most of these deaths. It was a veritable slaughter that no military machine could ever hope to equal. Most of those millions of deaths were due to heroic dosage and "plenty of good, nourishing food to keep up strength."

The records of recoveries and the much lower death rates under Christian science, Osteopathy, Chiropractic, Naturopathy, etc., reveal the true cause of death. "Killed by his (or her) physician" should have been carved on the tomb stones of practically all who died.

At present the sulfa drugs are being used. The country is full of people who are suffering from the effects of these drugs. They take these powerful poisons for colds, sore throats, "influenza," etc. They get well of these troubles, as has always been the case, but suffer for months and years from the drugs. Someday we will erect a monument to these victims of "medical science" and on that monument the victims of the "miracle drugs" will be prominently represented.

Whether the condition is diagnosed as a severe cold, as influenza, or as pneumonia, the first thing that should be done is to stop eating. Absolutely no food, but water, should be allowed to pass the patient's lips until the acute symptoms have subsided. No drugs of any kind should be resorted to.

Go to bed and rest. Keep warm. Rest, fasting, warmth, — these are the needs. Have plenty of fresh air in your room. Under these conditions you may lie in bed and get well in a short time with no complications and no sequels.

If you have a cough, don't take any "cough medicines" to check the cough.

If you have fever, don't take any anti-pyretics to reduce or "control" the fever.

If you have pain, don't take any pain-killers (anodynes) to "relieve" your pains.

—174—

If there is diarrhea, do not take anything to stop the diarrhea. If there is constipation, do not use saline, or other purges and do not employ enemas to force bowel action.

You don't need treatment. The fever, inflammation, coughing, etc., constitute the healing process. Just get out of their way and permit them to complete their work. Don't try to "aid nature." She doesn't need your puny aid — she only asks that you cease interfering.

Who's on a Diet?

Writing a few years ago in *Health and Life* (London), Edgar J. Saxon expressed the wish that "the word 'diet' could be forever oblitered from the English language". He added: "I shall do my best never to use it again."

What had got Mr. Saxon so "steamed up" over this little, inoffensive word? He says "At the London Health Center, where every day I converse with all sorts of people, the mischief of this dreadful word is brought home to me again and again. It suggests something severely restricted, dull, grim, appealing only to those afflicted souls who cannot be happy unless they are doing something unpleasant, but to all the jollier, wholesomer, life-loving folk forbidding and even ridiculous!"

We can well appreciate Mr. Saxon's antipathy to the word and the uses to which it is commonly put. We meet people who think that to "go on a diet" is to reduce weight, and others who think "diets" are for diabetic patients or for some other sick indiivdual whose physiology is crippled. To "diet" is to restrict oneself, or to eat unpalatable foods. It is to deny oneself the joys and pleasures of eating.

This, however, is no fault of the word. This attitude has grown out of a general misuse of the word. Mr. Saxon, himself, is guilty of misusing the word when he says it is "legitimate, perhaps, in professional work," and suggests that "It should refer solely to special regimens essential for the removal of ill-health". He complains that "it has crept over into everyday talk with as a dreadful

consequence, a widespread notion that Food Reform means a *diet*, one particular way of feeding,
when in fact it means nothing of the sort".

It is quite true that Food Reform does not
necessarily mean "one particular way of feeding"
for food reform can take place without altering
the way of feeding. For instance, one can discard
white bread for whole wheat and go on eating
his bread in the same old way, combined as badly as before and can overeat on wholewheat
bread as much as he previously overate on white
bread.

Food Reform takes place when one abandons
all denatured or processed foods and eats only
natural foods. Eating reform may and may not
accompany. Eating reform occurs only when one
learns to take his foods properly.

There need be nothing grim, unappealing,
dull or restricted about either food reform or eating reform. On the contrary either or both of
these may be made more attractive, pleasant,
enlivening and varied than the conventional denatured, overcooked, seasoned, and largely food-
less diet and dietary practices.

To return to my main theme, let me say that
regardless of what kind of food one eats, how it
is prepared, how much he eats and how he eats
it, he is on a diet. He is dieting. The word diet
does not mean a *restricted diet*; it does not mean
a *special diet*; it does not mean a *diet* prescribed
by a doctor or a dietitian. To *diet* is not to miss
the legitimate pleasures of eating or to restrict
oneself to the particular dietary notions and practices of an individual or a group.

To diet is simply to eat. Your diet is simply
your food. The Greek word *diaita* meant a dining room or a summer house, a way of life, referring especially to food and dress, a dwelling.
The French, *diete* and the Latin, *dieta* meant
"a mode of living, diet; a dining room, summer

house". The word is derived from an Aryan root meaning "to live". It has a close connection with the Aryan root of the word *vital*, also meaning "to live", also with the Aryan root for *bio*, also meaning "a way of life".

The word has an ancient and honorable pedigree, having its roots in the original tongue of the Indo-European peoples and an original meaning of which it need not be ashamed.

In modern English usage the word diet has the following meanings:

1.—What one habitually eats and drinks.

2.—Usual fare.

3.—Daily fare; victuals.

4.—Manner of feeding—a *frugal diet*.

5.—Course of food specifically selected or prescribed — a diet of nuts and hot water; *to put a patient on a special diet*.

6.—To regulate or restrict the food and drink.

7.—To take food and drink according to a regimen — *eat carefully or sparingly*.

Thus it will be seen that the word is broad enough in its meaning to cover any eating practice any one at any time and place may indulge in. Whether you eat carefully or haphazardly; plan your meals or eat whatever is in sight; select your foods or eat them indiscriminately; restrict yourself or consume an inclusive fare; eat frugally or gluttonously; follow the dictates of your own fancy and taste or the advise of a doctor or a dietitian, you are *dieting;* you are on a *diet*. Whether you derive pleasure from your food or pain, whether it nourishes or poisons you, you are on a diet.

When you hear someone exclaim: "No doctor is going to put me on a diet! I am going to eat what I want", or "I am not going to diet", you may know that this person does not know the real meaning of the word diet. He or she is on a *diet*. The only way you can stay off a *diet* is to fast—

abstain from eating. As you cannot do this indefinitely, you will, in a few days to three months or a little longer, be back on a diet again.

Since we have to diet to live, since we cannot live longer than a few months (and most of us not this long) without eating, does it not behoove us to give up our prejudices about *diet* and *dieting* and apply a little intelligence to our selection, preparation and combination of foods and our practices of eating these?

A lady once consulted a Natural Therapist. She said to him: "I hope you won't ask me to do a whole host of unnecessary things, otherwise I shall have no time for anything else".

He replied:

"You will not be asked to do anything that will take up any extra time. You have got to *live* in any case and all I shall ask you to do is to *live correctly*. For instance, we all have to think, exercise, eat, breathe, clothe, cleanse, relax, recreate, drink and sleep. These are the ten commandments of health, and they are things we must do for and by ourselves. At least, no one else can do them for us successfully, and they do not require any more time to do them correctly. If they are undertaken in time and in the right spirit, they will bring the reward of better health".

I can well appreciate the woman's fear that she would be asked to do a lot of unnecessary and time-consuming things. I once took all the things its readers were advised to do daily in only one issue of a popular health magazine and estimated the time that would be required to carry them all out as instructed. I found they would consume the whole day and leave no time for anything else. *Unfortunately*, some of us have to work in addition to looking after our health — a thing many of our contemporaries have not learned.

Time is a valuable asset in life, and by the right use of it, and especially what is called leisure time, health may be promoted and maintained. But the important fact is that it requires no more time to live correctly than it does to live incorrectly. Indeed, correct living usually saves time. It requires no more time to eat wholesome food in proper combinations than it does to eat unwholesome foods in improper combinations. It requires less time to prepare foods properly than improperly. The only person who might lose any time in eating correctly is the person who has been in the habit of bolting his food. He'll require more time to thoroughly chew it. This will compensate him, however, by increasing his enjoyment of food and by relieving him of his abdominal distress.

It requires less time to eat moderately than to eat gluttonously. As moderate eating is also more economical and more healthful the advantages are all on the side of moderation. Moderate eating is not a "restricted diet" except in the sense that all healthful, wholesome and pleasurable activities have their limitations beyond which they become unhealthful, unwholesome and unpleasant.

Since we must eat to live and are, therefore on a diet at all times, except on those rare occasions when some of us fast, it behooves us to exercise enough intelligence in our feeding habits to guarantee that we are on a healthful diet. We can derive as much, or more, pleasure from a wholesome diet as from an unwholesome one without the troublesome pathological consequences of the latter. It is only unintelligent dieting that we should fear. It is a diet made up of unwholesome substances that we should shun. We will not be hurt if, in our eating habits, we use our heads for something besides hat-racks.

Mr. Saxon suggests substituting the rather bulky and awkward term "honest food" for the word diet. I have no fault to find with honesty but I don't like this unwieldly term. By "honest food" he simply means whole-foods — unprocessed and unadulterated. He says: "Let us return to honest foods, then we shall not go a-whoring after paraffin, glucose and roughage." This is sound advice and we approve.

We also approve when he says: "Food reform begins and ends with discrimination, choice and pleasure. Abstinence from unwholesome food is not a good beginning, and it is a very bad end. Abstinence is healthy only when it easily and inevitably results from choice of something better."

The emphasis should be placed on the positive side — on the side of wholesomeness, integrity, pleasure and fitness to supply the needs of the body; not on the negative side — that of mere abstinence from unwholesome foods, as essential as this is.

Mr. Saxon also attempts to destroy what he calls "the stuffy old British bogey 'plain food'." He says: "People occasionally tell me they have always preferred 'plain food.' Often, alas, their looks support the statement. For during the past fifty years what has 'plain food' usually meant? It has meant white bread, white sugar, boiled suet pudding with golden syrup (golden! How deep an iniquity to debase that resplendent sun-lit word to the description of a sticky and un-natural 'refinement' of honest sugar-cane juice!); sloppy sweetened porridge that slithers past the teeth, milk puddings made of sham rice that produces physical decay in Oriental people; taste-less ruined vegetables with their essential value enriching the drains; starchy pea soup; sour fruit cooked with white sugar; cocoa (or drink for life-despisers); cornflour blancmange (a form of stickphast); meat gravy and meat extracts (akin to urine in content); Marie and Petit-Beurre biscuits (why did they give pretty French names to such futile products?); forty-horsepower Indian tea that tans the innards and bloats or withers the human form divine; lemonade crystals and powders that have caught only a fleeting glance from an honest lemon; potted chicken and duck deriving from bacon factories; custard powder that has no milk in it and never has seen a honest bird laying an egg. This is your 'plain food' in practice — one vast, insidious, devastating curse."

America's dietary practices are not identical with those of the British but are sufficiently like them that the above description of the "plain foods" of the people over there needs but little change to fit our practices over here. There is really an urgent need for a return to honest foods — to foods that are what they pretend to be and not denatured and adulterated products such as are eaten three times a day on most of the tables throughout the length of our land.

The daintiest dinner can conform to an honest base. But, as Mr. Saxon points out, "honest food need not be 'plain' unless you desire it." The ingenuity of the average wife and mother may easily turn the simplest fare into a festival without either spoiling the food or violating the rules of proper food combining.

"Neither is Food Reform faddy," says Mr. Saxon. "A fad is an end symptom of spiritual disorder, and in so far as the Food Reform 'movement' has produced a horde of faddists it is open to drastic condemnation." Unless the exercise of common intelligence in making use of the store of knowledge man has gained is a fad, food reform is not a fad. Unless it is a fad to be healthy, food reform, that is, healthful eating

is not a fad. But if the unthinking multitude ·
continues to look upon sanity in the choice, preparation and eating of food as a fad let it
think so; it is still better to be a healthy faddist
than a sick and dying scientist. Govern not your
life by what fools say and think.

Rat-Pen Dietetics

Recently I read a magazine article by a woman who was proud of the fact that she had grown big children, though she seems not to have asked herself if, perchance, they were not too big. Her boy was ten and as large as the average fourteen year old. This size she attributed to her program of feeding, which, up to school age, consisted of feeding every three hours by the clock.

Precocious development may easily be brought about by nutritive redundancy, but there is plenty of evidence that it is undesirable. There is also every reason to believe that moderate degrees of giantism result in lowered resistance, lessened fertility and shortened life. But I do not write this article to discuss a subject that I am preparing a fuller discussion of for future publication. I desire, rather, to call attention to another fallacy contained in her article.

She mentions what "men of science" have done with the sizes of guinea pigs in their experimental work with diets and asks: "Why could this not apply also to our children." Then she says:

"Comparing pigs to children isn't so strange. Scientists use the guineas in their laboratory experiments not only because they are so prolific and therefore easily obtainable, but because they are most nearly like the human being and susceptible to most of the ailments that affect humans."

The fallacy in that statement lies in the assertion that guinea pigs are "most nearly like the human being." There are many animals that more closely resemble man in structure and function than does the guinea pig. But none of them are identical with man and none of them give results in experiments that are identical with the results of the same experiments in man.

The fact is that, while there is a fundamental unity in all animal life, from amoeba to man, there are specific differences, even between closely related species, that make animal experiments often misleading. There is only one experiment that can be relied upon in man and this is performed on man, not on guinea pigs or rats.

The last experiment must always be upon man, testified Professor Starling before the British Royal Commission Investigating Vivisection. Why? Because what works on animals does not always work on man.

Medicine is proud of the fact that it is "scientific." It proves the *value* of all of its *cures* by the "scientific method" — that is, the experimental method. But the careful observer cannot fail to see that after the "scientific method" has fully established the value of a new (or an old) cure, the "unscientific method"— that is, the empirical method — rapidly proves that it not only does not cure, but actually damages and kills patients. Since no "scientific" physician would admit that he is a mere empiricist, he dignifies the old empirical method by calling it the *clinical method*. Call it what you will, after the laboratory has shown the new remedy to be good, bedside experience proves it to be bad.

Some of my readers may recall when physiologists experimented on the brains of animals in an effort to locate the brain centers in the human brain. They could not find a "mathematics center" in the ape and decided man does not have one. Such is the misleading tendency of some experiments.

Pharmacologists follow, literally, the old advice to "try it on the dog" and try out their drugs on various kinds of animals. They long ago discovered that the same drug induced or provoked different reaction in different kinds of animals. The only way they can determine what action it will occasion in man is by trying it out on man.

A pigeon can take enough morphine to kill several men and fly away as though nothing happened. Hogs can take enough prussic acid to kill many men, with no apparent harm. Rabbits grow fat on belladonna, but if we included it in the salads fed our children, we would soon be without children.

What is known as the "biological test" in feeding, that is, trying it out on the dog, turns out as much fallacy as trying out drugs on the dogs. I have often wondered what the "biologists" would feed us if they used sewer rats as experimental animals. If they were to use buzzards in their experiments they would discover that rotting meat from a hog that had died of cholera is good food. Dogs eat bones and digest them with case. It is doubtful that man could get away with a bone diet so easily. Tobacco worms live on tobacco — you try it, worm.

Anything we desire to prove can be proved on the lower animals if we only use a sufficient number of kinds of animals. Rat-pen (or guinea pig) dietetics has simply led the dietitians astray in more ways than one. They have worked out their solutions to human problems in their test tubes, guinea pigs and rats, and not in the human body. As a consequence, they do not even know dietetics.

It would be folly to say their animal experimentation has not provided some knowledge or that it has not supplied leads that have been useful, but the tendency is to rely too much on the results of the animal experiments in feeding men, women and children.

Always Eating —
Always Hungry

A man sends me a diet program prescribed for him by a Naturopath and says the doctor said that "in between meals I could have as much fruits as I wanted, providing I am hungry and I am always hungry."

Following out this program, which was prescribed for a particular heart affection, he developed one of those famous "attacks" that we are constantly reading and hearing about. He was examined by a medical man who told him his "attack" was due to overeating.

When a man eats enough that a medical man tells him that he overeats, he must really be eating a lot of food. In fact, I judge from the man's report that he ate practically all day.

Eating all the time and *always* hungry! How is it possible? It is not possible. This man, like most men, has mistaken morbid irritation of his stomach for hunger. The constant eating has only perpetuated and intensified the irritation.

We have got to get over the foolish idea that so long as we eat fruits we can eat all we want at any and all times of the day (and night) under any condition of life and in any combination we please.

This continued eating, this putting fruit into a stomach already full of other foods in the process of digestion, results in the souring of food in the digestive tract. The digestive tract goes into the business of manufacturing vinegar, alcohol and gas. There is no better way of getting sick than eating of this type.

The patient complains of much gas with frequent passing of gas. He says it has a very foul odor. Also he complains that frequent desires to go to stool turn out to be false alarms. He passes only gas.

What does all this mean? Simply this: *indigestion* with *fermentation* and rectal *irritation*. Sooner or later he will begin to pass mucus and not merely gas. He will find himself suffering with colitis. All of this trouble arises largely (not wholly) out of overeating.

Perhaps the Naturopath who attempted to direct this man's eating did not tell him to eat at all times of the day and night. If he told him to eat when hungry, he did not mean that every morbid sensation the man experienced was to be mistaken for hunger.

I believe in always eating when hungry and never eating when not hungry. But I long ago learned that this advise is dangerous when given to the food addict. The addict is, as this man says of himself, "always hungry." This is to say, he thinks he is always hungry—though, in reality, he is never hungry. His trouble is that he has not learned to distinguish between the symptoms of disease and the normal demand of the body for nourishment.

Eating, with these people, has degenerated into a habit — a morbid habit. They are constantly trying to appease a voracious monster that can be appeased only by denying him gratification. The more he is fed, the more he demands. The more food is consumed, the more voracious grows the appetite.

These people cannot be trusted to eat when hungry. To advise them to do so is to defeat the very purpose of the advice. They need a prolonged period of abstinence to relieve them of most, at least, of their morbid cravings and their symptoms which they persist in mistaking for hunger.

After this, they need a prolonged period of education and guidance. For, eating habits are mental as well as physical. It is as important to educate them out of their faulty mental habits as to educate them out of faulty physical habits. It will be best for these people to get away entirely from their present environment and all of its associations and cultivate and firmly establish new habits before returning home. Most of them are too weak to succeed in any other way.

Food Cures

The belief in *cures* is so old and so deeply grounded in the intellectual heritage of our people that even men who should know better talk of *cures* and of the *therapeutic* value of things that are used as *cures*. These men, although they do not believe in drug *cures*, find it easy to believe in food *cures*. Certain foods are said to possess certain *therapeutic* or *curative* powers. Some of these foods have been used for ages as *cures* and the superstition is hard to down.

In this article we shall discuss the superstitions that cluster around the onion family — onions, scallions or shallots, leeks, garlic, and chives. It would be difficult to say how old is the belief in the curative properties of these substances, a belief that seems to have grown out of their sharp "taste" which is really irritation caused by the mustard oil they contain.

"All strong tasting foods are usually believed to have curative powers," says one author, while discussing garlic. "For instance," he says, "all sharp tasting foods are supposed to have blood-cleansing properties." Although radishes belong to the mustard, rather than to the onion, family, hence do not properly belong in this discussion, it will not be amiss to point out that, due to their mustard oil content, they have the same sharp "taste" as the onion family and have long been thought to possess curative powers. In ancient times black radishes were thought "to have specific therapeutic value in treating gallstones." The juice was extracted from one radish by pounding it, and then mixed with white wine or grape juice and taken once a day. Today the radish is said to be a "stimulant of the digestive tract."

Let us now address ourselves to the food plants that we propose to consider in this article. We shall take them up in alphabetical order.

Chives contain a large amount of mustard oil which gives them their sharp "taste". They are claimed to "stimulate the appetite, help secrete the gastric juices by stimulating the digestive organs", and "exercise a strong diuretic effect." They are referred to as "digestive stimulants, exciting the flow of saliva and gastric juice." They are said to "aid in dissolving phlegm in catarrh." Because of their *strong diuretic action,* "it is commonly believed that these vegetables are particularly beneficial as a blood cleanser."

Garlic is also rich in mustard oil. It is claimed to be a "digestive stimulant." It strongly stimulates the appetite and acid secretions of the gastric juices and so prevents flatulency or gas formation." Speaking of the belief that "all sharp tasting foods have blood cleansing properties" the above quoted author says: "in a sense this does apply to garlic."

It is said to have "anti-bacterial action" and is often referred to as a "germ-killer." It contains a substance called *crotonaldehyde* that is said to be a bactericide. For this reason, garlic is said to be particularly excellent for "bacterial diseases" of the nose and respiratory tract. It is also often referred to as an "intestinal antiseptic" and is frequently recommended for the eradication of intestinal parasites and "recently has been prescribed for singers and speakers." It is "furthermore said to be helpful in gout, inflammation of the trachea, asthma, and even in tuberculosis. Many physicians are said to have used it with good results in cases of pulmonary consumption." Because of "its iodine content, it is also useful in treating goitre." It is also recommended and used in cases of high blood pressure and in cases of arterial calcination.

It has a diuretic action" and "aids in destroying stones." "Although its diuretic action has been proven, garlic juice because of its mustard oil content is very irritating to the kidneys."

Leeks contain a small amount of mustard oil. They are said to "share the germicidal property of the entire onion group." We learn that "bowls of leek soup known centuries ago as treatment for colds and laryngitis," while "the Roman Emperor Nero used leeks therapeutically to clear his voice." They are "recommended for inflammation of the air passages and for colds because they tend to loosen phlegm and to cure a cough." They "may be given alone or in soup, to help relieve colds or other respiratory infections." They are "beneficial" in treating gout, rheumatism, gall stones and heart pains.

Leeks "stimulate the action of the salivary and digestive glands and increase the appetite." They are also "noted for their power in promoting urine secretions and in preventing flatulency."

Onions vary in their content of ethereal mustard oil. "Recent experiments indicate that onion fumes contain a therapeutic agent called allyl aldehyde. Chemical enters the blood; can kill germs and viruses."

They "are recommended for colds, hoarsness, coughs, catarrh dizziness (vertigo), dropsy, dysuria, loss of appetite, body and breast pains, flatulency, constipation, face aches, headaches, murmurings in the ears, worms, etc."

They have long been used as a "digestant" and to "encourage contractions of stomach and stimulate flow of gastric juices." We are informed that "a small roasted onion was often given in European sanitaria after each meal to aid digestion." They are also said to be "strongly diuretic in their action."

There was an old belief that onions were good in curing baldness. They are "also believed today to aid insomniacs, in sleeping. A raw onion sandwich or a bowl of onion soup before retiring may help bring sleep easily."

We are advised by another author that it is "best to use onions cooked in soup rather than raw for therapeutic purposes."

Scallions or shallots are small plants belonging to the onion family. Not much seems to be claimed for them, though we are assured that they "share the germicidal property of the entire onion group." One author tells us that the entire onion family (onions, chives, leeks, garlic, scallions, etc.) is "known therapeutically as a bactericide" and "is particularly good for infections of the nose and throat; Beneficial (when made into soup) for warding off and relieving colds."

The reader will note that the claims made for each of these foods have much in common. It will be best to discuss these common attributes first.

All of them are said to stimulate the appetite. If this is true, they induce overeating and, in this particular, have a harmful influence. There is never a time or condition of life when appetite should be stimulated. If there is lack of desire for food this is because there is no need for food or no ability to digest and absorb it. It is best to wait for hunger.

All of them are said to stimulate the flow of the digestive juices. It should be understood that all true digestive juices contain one or more enzymes. The pouring out of an enzymeless juice to lubricate a food or to dilute an irritating substance and help to wash it away does not aid digestion. It should also be known that the digestive

juice adapted to the digestion of an onion would not be adapted to the digestion of bread or meat.

They are said to increase the flow of acid gastric juice. This would be a distinct hindrance to the digestion of starches. It is just what one should seek to avoid. On the other hand, an excess of acid actually retards protein digestion and if the excess is great enough stops it altogether.

The informed reader will understand that the increased secretion occasioned by the eating of these foods is due to their irritating effects. The secretions are intended to dilute and wash away the irritation. These secretions are mixed with much mucus.

They are said to promote peristalsis. This is also the result of their irritating effect. The increased action of the digestive tract is intended to move them along more rapidly and get rid of them. After toleration is established this action ceases. There follows, then, a slowing down of peristalsis.

We can't goad and prick the organs of the body with any substance and expect them to function normally. Such treatment always produces weakness.

We may safely say that the use of these foods does not improve digestion, does not prevent or relieve flatulency, does not prevent or cure constipation, and does not cure inflammation of the digestive tract. The large numbers of people who suffer with these very conditions and who eat these foods regularly is proof enough that these *cures* do not cure.

They are all said to be germ killers and are, therefore, recommended in "infections," but especially in respiratory "infections", that is, in such catarrhal conditions as colds, bronchitis, laryngitis, asthma, cough, etc. They are said not only to kill germs in these conditions, but to loosen and dissolve phlegm (mucus).

Their germ-killing potency is very small as it does not even protect them against bacterial action. That they frequently decompose in the digestive tract is well known.

They do not loosen mucus. The body merely pours out much thin, watery mucus to dilute and wash away the irritating juices and fumes of these foods.

That they neither cure nor prevent the respiratory diseases they are said to cure and "ward off" is apparent to all who will use their eyes. Look around you and see the millions who suffer with these very conditions and who use these foods regularly.

They are all said to have "diuretic action". This means they increase urination. But the action is not the action of the onion family. It is the action of the kidneys. The kidneys increase their action to aid the body in removing the irritating qualities of these foods from the body. The increased urination following their use is not due to their beneficial effects but to their harmful properties. Try dropping a little onion juice in your eye and try to convince yourself that the burning and smarting thus produced is beneficial. There will be a profuse flow of tears; not because the onion juice benefits the eyes, but because it irritates them and the tears are intended to dilute and wash away the irritating juice.

They are all said to be blood purifiers. This is an old superstition. There are but few blood purifiers and these are all in the body. We know them as the liver, kidneys, lungs, colon and a few glands. If we judge the onions by the ways the body handles them, we should conclude that they befoul the blood.

Most, if not all of them, are said to prevent and cure gall stones. I need devote no more space to this claim than the little that is required to say they do neither of these things.

When the behaviour of the body towards a food substance is the same as its behaviour towards drugs, this does not mean that the food has the same beneficial effects long mistakenly attributed to these poisons; but that there is some harmful substance in the food, which, like the drug, must be promptly eliminated to prevent harm. In the case of members of the onion family, the mustard oil they contain irritates not only the mouth and digestive tract, but the kidneys and, perhaps, all parts of the body with which it come in contact. It is not likely that this irritation of the digestive tract and kidneys can be long continued without doing harm.

These things are eaten regularly for the same reason that salt, pepper, spices, mustard, horse radish, etc., are eaten. They are used as condiments and are especially relished by men and women of perverted taste. So fond are they of the sharp "taste" of these foods, they will eat them even when going to church, the theater or elsewhere, where the foul breath they produce will annoy others.

From observations of patients I suspect that their habitual use is often partly responsible for degenerative forms of nervous diseases. I certainly cannot advise their regular use and would say that, at best, they are foods to be used on rare occasions.

Food Cures (Cont.)

Among the many delightful fruits with which the plant kingdom tempts its animal partners, one of the most luscious and healthful is the papaya. Marco Polo is credited with having discovered this fruit, which he described as a strange, tropical melon and he credited it with having *cured* his sailors of scurvy. After Polo's discovery the fruit was found growing in various parts of the tropics — India, the South Sea Islands, the West Indies, and elsewhere.

Six hundred or more edible fruits are grown in the world today and the papaya is classed among the first ten of these. It is our opinion that the basis of these classifications is faulty and we do not take them seriously. Fruits are food, not "medicines"; they nourish the body and do not *cure* it.

In the United States this delicious fruit is grown in Florida, California and the Rio Grande Valley of Texas. The tree grows rapidly and bears fruit early, beginning to bear in ten months after the seeds are planted. As it bears continuously, the crop lasts throughout the year. Fortunate are those folk who live where this fruit may be picked fully ripened from the tree.

Like most fruits, the papaya is valuable chiefly for its minerals and vitamins. Analyses of the fruit show that it contains appreciable percentages of iron, potassium, phosphorus, manganese, silicon, sodium, calcium, sulphur, magnesium and aluminum. Minerals are present in fruits in the form of organic salts and are readily assimilated by the body.

The vitamin content of the papaya is a feature that has attracted considerable attention. *Bulletin No.* 77 of the Department of Agriculture tells us that the papaya contains four vitamins. The vitamin content, according to International units per 100 gms., is about 2,500 units of vitamin A, 33 units of Vitamin B, and 70 units of Vitamin C. Vitamin D is present but undetermined. This is a relatively high vitamin content.

The *Review* recommends the papaya to all who can obtain it as a food and not as a digestant, not as a cure, not as a cosmetic. It is our opinion that too much fuss has been made about the fact that it is the only known vegetable source of *papain*, or what is often called vegetable pepsin.

Papain is remarkably similar to the pepsin found in the human stomach and has similar catalytic effects upon proteins. Unlike all animal pepsins, it is said to act in any digestive medium — neutral, alkaline or acid. Animal pepsins act only in acid mediums.

The presence of this enzyme in the papaya has caused it to be prescribed in cases of impaired digestion. The papain is said to help digest protein foods — flesh of all kinds, milk, eggs, etc. If it actually has this effect, there is still no reason why it should be prescribed for impaired digestion and there are good reasons why it should not be so prescribed.

The use of "digestants" never corrects or removes the causes of impaired digestion. The use of papain instead of the pepsin of the drugstore (taken from the stomach of a hog) is only another effort to cure disease without removing its cause. The use of either substance is based on the same false principle.

There is evidence that when pepsin is taken with meals it causes our own pepsin-secreting glands to depend on the outside source and to lay down on the job. They are injured by this *crutch* and, if the injury is great, do not fully recover. It is probable that the use of papain in the same way produces the same effect.

It is always best to depend on your own physiological powers to do your own physiological work and not rely upon crutches. The papaya should, therefore, be eaten alone or at a fruit meal and should not be taken with proteins. If digestion is impaired, do not impair it further by resort to a crutch; but remove the cause of the impairment and give the digestive system sufficient rest to restore normal secretion.

The papaya is claimed to do other work that it probably does not do. It is claimed to assist in the conversion of starches and sugars to levulose and dextrose and thus "relieve" the digestive glands of overwork. Pepsin does not act upon carbohydrates, but if there are other enzymes in the papaya that do, there are the same objections to the employment of such crutches as there are to the use of papain. The best way to avoid overwork of the digestive glands is not to overeat.

Therapeutic effects are claimed for the use of the papaya that make it rival sulfanilamide as a near cure-all. No intelligent and informed person will be misled by the so-called "clinical" results obtained from the use of this very fine fruit. It is very unfortunate that no good fruit can be used as a food, but must be presented to us as a marvelous cure for many of our ills. Food-drugs are hawked on every hand.

The papaya is said to be a normalizer: it "promotes" the generation and flow of the salivary and gastric juices as much as four and five times in some cases, reduces excess gastric acidity, relieves flatulence and the pain resulting from excess gas, reduces mucus in the stomach, intestine and colon to a thin liquid that is easily disposed of, and soothes and heals the irritated areas of the digestive tract. These are only part of the curative effects attributed to the papaya.

Its external use is said to dissolve the false membrane of diphtheria, to relieve skin irritations such as eczema, sunburn and poison ivy. As a cosmetic it is claimed to contain an enzyme that tends to "bring out the live tissue, giving a fresh youthful effect."

Watch this fruit. Other, perhaps, even more marvelous claims will be made for it. As it is, we are assured that its "proven" health benefits are numerous and amazing, while "research" is being carried on in many places to find its other hidden magics. After all is said about the papaya, it is also one of the most delicious fruits known to man and the statement that in the natural state its flavor, while not unpleasant, is definitely not appealing, can be made only by those who have never eaten this fruit. It is one of our finest fruits — a fine food — to be recommended to all who can get it.

The bottled juices of the papaya that are on the market and the other papaya products that are offered to the public may be good food substances, but they lack the fine flavor of the fresh, tree-ripened papaya, and the claims made that these products are superior in taste and value to nature's unchanged product are all, without exception, false. Such claims can be made seriously only by those who have never tasted a fresh, ripe papaya.

Vitamin Failures

Writing in the August 1943 issue of *The Health Walker*, Ned Zane tells of a little incident that occurred on one of the hikes at the recent convention of the International Hikers, held in West Virginia.

He tells of a doctor who, "on the day we hiked to Lloydsville, Ohio, was taking vitamin tablets and passed them around to others."

Eating "vitamin" tablets is a very common folly today. We are advised to eat them for energy, for health, to prevent disease, to cure disease, to enable us to get drunk without harm and for a lot of other things. This vitamin-eating doctor should have been in the pink of condition. He should have been full of energy and endurance. Mr. Zane says of him:

"But he could not make the grade from Blaine to Saint Clairsville, and had to abandon the hike. All the girls beat him. This is a striking example of what all these vitamin pills and capsules are worth."

It will be objected that one such experience is not conclusive proof. We grant this and if this were the only evidence of the worthlessness of these pills we would not bother to repeat Zane's account of the incident.

Mr. Zane truly adds: "The old-time patent medicine crowd are making millions of dollars on them (vitamin pills) at the expense of poor dupes among the public." Profits from these newer frauds are not, of course, confined to the old patent-medicine crowd. Even the soap manufacturers are now in the game manufacturing "vitamins."

"It would appear" says Mr. Zane, "to be the duty of the medical profession to expose these frauds; but do they do it? Does the American Medical Association do it?"

It is wrong to think or assume that the medical profession or the American Medical Association has a "duty". This profession exists to further its own profits. Its association was formed to increase the power and profits of the profession. Why should it expose the patent-medicine crowd? The medical profession and the patent-medicine crowd are one and the same and must "sink or swim, survive or perish" together.

Ask the medical profession to expose these fraudulent vitamins! The profession is prescribing them in ever increasing amounts. Physicians, themselves, are taking them. They are giving them to their children the same as to their patients. How can a profession that is so ignorant that it is "taken in" by this fraud be expected to expose it.

Mr. Zane next says: "The best way to get the necessary vitamins is to eat our food raw, as in salads. Take them fresh from the trees or the ground, wash them and eat them before they have time to wilt. Ordinary cooking destroys vitamins to the extent of about 25% to 40%; and cooking in autoclave or pressure cooker destroys them about 100%. So, to avoid illness for yourself and your family, you must avoid all such foods including all canned foods thus preserved. Dr. Paul Carton says: 'The pressure cooker is the graveyard of the vitamins'."

Dr. Carton is a famous French physician and scientist who has partially abandoned drugs and has gone a long way into the Nature Cure or Hygienic field. He was formerly (and may yet be) head of a famous tubercular sanitarium near Paris. He has made considerable study of food and knows a little about the subject.

What he says about the pressure cooker being the graveyard of the vitamins is true. Cooking foods under high presssure is one of the worst, if not the worst, forms of cooking now employed. It is safe to say that all cooking is bad — some modes of cooking are merely less damaging than others.

Natural foods contain more than an ample supply of all the known and unknown vitamins needed by human and animal life. There is no need for resort to *phoney* vitamins from the drug store or the five-and-ten.

Natural foods supply man, as they do the wild horse or the deer, with all the nutritive elements needed for normal growth, an abundance of energy, great strength, endurance, reproductive power and resistance against the unfavorable influences and agents in our environment. These foods do not need the chemist, nor the food manufacturer to aid them in supplying all the nutritive materials essential to superior nutrition. Vitamin pills do not belong to natural living.

. . . .

. . . .
. . . .
. . . .

. . . .
. . . .

Are There
Mucus-Forming Foods?

Let us get it straight: there is no such thing as a *mucus-forming* food. For several years, now, this idea that there are mucus forming and non-mucus forming foods has been troubling the people of this country. The idea seems to have been originated by the late Arnold Ehret.

Ehret, it seems, was a German veterinarian who fled his homeland when the World War broke out in 1914. Going first to Switzerland, he finally found his way to America where he remained until he died at a not advanced age. He posed as a nature curist and claimed knowledge and experience he did not have. He preached principles he did not follow, claimed a state of health he did not possess, and was responsible for much fallacy in the health movement.

He not only classified foods as mucus forming and non-mucus forming, he did not know the difference between mucus and pus. He posed as an authority on fasting, yet when challenged by Dr. Linda Burfield Hazzard at a public lecture, admitted from the platform that his experience with fasting was almost none. He is the inventor of that widely sold mixture of dried herbs that sells under the trade name of *Inner Clean*.

Mucus is made (secreted) by the cells (mucus-glands) of the mucous membrane lining all the hollow organs of the body that communicate either directly or indirectly with the outside world. Mucus is secreted by these membranes in the healthiest individual living in the most ideal manner under the best conceivable environments.

It is the normal lubricant of these surfaces, keeping them moist and preventing cracking and drying. In the bronchial tubes it assists in carrying dust out of the lungs. If irritants get into the nose it is secreted in quantity to aid in expelling these. If irritants or poisons get into the stomach, intestine and colon, large quantities of mucus are poured out to dilute these and flush them away.

Mucus is a normal physiological product serving definite and useful functions in the body. It is produced by the "mucous cells" from materials supplied them by the blood. Blood is the "mucus forming" material. Mucus does not float around in the blood to be expelled at some point or other in the body.

In catarrh, which is inflammation (acute or chronic) of the mucous membrane, there is an excess of mucus, of thick, ropy, discolored character. Excess of foods, especially of carbohydrate foods, helps to produce and maintain the catarrhal condition. Acetous fermentation resulting from excess starch, sugar and fat eating, produces toxins that are eliminated through the mucous membrane in the form of catarrh.

These foods do not form mucus, they form acids when they ferment. Eating when digestion is temporarily inhibited permits fermentation to take place. The formation of acids, like the formation of mucus, is the work of cells, of bacteria.

Foods left to themselves and not acted upon by organized ferments (bacteria) or unorganized ferments (enzymes) remain, just about the same. They don't form anything. They are merely materials out of which things are formed.

ARE THERE MUCUS-FORMING FOODS?

Food excess, even excesses of those foods classed by Ehret as non-mucus forming, may result in catarrh or may increase it; not because foods are mucus forming, but because the body often rids itself of acids and excesses by forming these into mucus. If so-called mucus forming foods are not eaten in excess of the body's power to digest and utilize them, no catarrhal trouble results therefrom.

It is possible to overeat on the best of foods. I know there are those who doubt this, but such are either inexperienced or blind. Overeating is a frequent cause of indigestion. Indigestion is only another term for fermentation. For when the unorganized ferments (enzymes) are inadequate for the work of digestion, the organized ferments (bacteria) take over the work of breaking down and dissolving the food. The products of the two processess are very unlike each other. One of them prepares food for use by the body, the other renders it unfit for use.

Indigestion products, when these find their way into the blood stream, must be eliminated. Catarrh is one of the means of eliminating these toxic matters.

Tables of Food Analysis

For years we have told people that tables and charts giving the chemical analyses foods are only play-things for the laboratory boys; that for the man in the street, or even for the doctor in his office or at the bed-side, they have no practical value. Any man or woman who attempted to plan a dietary on the basis of these analyses and to carry out such a dietary would either give up in disgust, or go crazy on the subject.

Since the discovery of vitamins it is all the more evident that these tables of food analysis are not of value. Prior to that discovery it was known that the tables, even if they could be assumed to be accurate (and they never are), could not show the digestibility of foods, nor could they reveal the capacity of the eater to appropriate what they contain.

I recall reading an article by Dr. Harvey W. Wiley, about pie. This article was published in *Good Housekeeping* back in the days before we first made the world safe for democracy. Referring to the chemical analysis of pies the doctor remarked (I quote from memory): "The food value of pie is not doubted; it only remains (or requires) to be digested."

There are few things that are more indigestible than pie, and despite their richness in food value, as shown by chemical analysis, the man who eats pies does not receive the expected nourishment from them.

Many years ago prof. Thomas Henry Huxley wrote about tables of food analysis: "It may be worth while to point out here that mere chemical analysis is, by itself, a very insufficient guide as to the usefulness and nutritive value of an article of food. A substance to be nutritious must not only contain some or other of the above food-stuffs, but contain them in ·an available, that is, digestible form. A piece of beef-steak is far more nourishing than a quantity of pease-pudding containing even a larger proportion of proteid material because the former is far more digestible than the altter. And a small piece of dry, hard cheese, though of high nutritive value as judged by mere chemical analysis, will not satisfy the more subtle criticism of the stomach."

There is a gross error in Prof. Huxley's statement above. He asumes, as does almost everyone else, that the nutritive value of a food is determined, to a large degree, by what they call its digestibility. It is, of course, true that if a food is not digested it yields up no nourishment; but this is not what he means when he says a food is more digestible or less digestible than another. He is referring, rather, to what is meant by the terms "hard" to digest and "easy" to digest.

With the exceptions of beans, peas, lentils and cereals, there are no foods that are "hard" to digest. There was in the days when Prof. Huxley graced the physiological profession, and is now, the tendency to determine the digestibility of a food by the time it remains in the stomach. We now know, even if we ignore it, that this time is determined, not by the ease or difficulty of digestion, but by the nature of the digestive process required to digest a particular food. A food that digests in the stomach in four hours is not necessarily more difficult to digest and does not demostrably use up more energy in being digested, than one that digests in one hour. The digestive process is simply different.

Readers who desire a knowledge of the processes of digestion so that they may more fully understand the above facts, should study Volume two of the *Hygienic System*.

Those vegetarians who would be more appropriately called "cerealists", that is, those who drop meat from their diet and substitute large quantities of cereals therefor, usually do so, because they are told that whole wheat, for instance, is an almost perfect food — "has all the elements the body needs in about the right proportions." These people not only consume too much starch, for which they suffer, but they eat their cereals in forms that tend to ferment before they digest.

Look for instance, at the gooey dish of boiled oat-meal to which has been added milk and sugar, so commonly eaten. It is one of the worst abominations that ever slipped down the human throat. It is practically indigestible. No saliva and no ptyalin are poured out upon such a dish and it may remain in the stomach for hours, undergoing little or no digestion, before it is allowed to pass into the intestine. Fermentation is inevitable. Cracked wheat, soaked, boiled and served with milk and sugar, milk and honey, milk and sweet fruits, is equally as indigestible.

The oatmeal or cracked wheat, or any other soaked or boiled cereal does not undergo salivary digestion, even when and if eaten without milk and sugar. When eaten in the usual combination, digestion is doubly impossible.

Flake cereal foods (various types of corn-flakes and other such foods) are much in use. Chemical analysis shows them to be possessed of abundant food value, though, actually they are largely charcoal. They are said to be ready-cooked and predigested. This is a fallacy that the public must outgrow. They are pressed between rollers at intense heat and are rendered practically valueless as foods.

Chemical analysis of canned foods will show them to possess practically all the food value contained in the original or 'fresh food before it underwent the canning process. Feeding tests reveal that they have lost much of their value.

Canned milks are shown, by chemical analysis, to be concentrated foods. They actually contain more food value, pound for pound, than fresh milk. Feeding tests show that while an animal or child will live, thrive and grow on fresh, whole, raw milk, the same animal or child will sicken and die on canned milk.

It is well to know that a complete analysis of the human body has never been made and no complete analyses of all food substances have ever been made. Even if food tables could be of practical use to the man-in-the-street, they would be very misleading in our present state of knowledge of the chemistry of the body.

What we have said about tables of food chemistry applies equally to vitamin charts. For example, it is claimed that under certain conditions of vitamin deficiency, feeding a diet abundant in the deficient vitamin often fails to help, because the patient fails to assimilate the vitamins in the diet.

In such cases efforts are made to supply vitamins by injecting them into the blood stream. We are told that "Reliance, therefore, cannot be placed in the mere presence of vitamins and of other requisite elements in the diet."

The value of any food, under any condition, is not determined wholly by its chemical composition and its vitamin content, but largely by the ability of the body to extract from it and make use of the nourishment it contains. Contrary to medical theory and practice, the body is not a machine that is capable of utilizing a certain amount of food at all times and under all conditions.

When to Eat

Old superstitions die hard. Some Irishman is reported to have said that they have to be "repeatedly killed." This would seem to be so, at least, if we can assume that they are ever really killed. It seems to me they never die.

Just now I have in mind some old superstitions about eating that were exploded over a hundred years ago by Sylvester Graham, re-exploded about forty-five to fifty years ago by Dr. Dewey, and are still with us, still doing "business as usual."

One of those monthly almanacs issued by the "health food" trade, recently came to my desk. In it is presented a "Dipsy Diet" for reducing. The daily menus provide for five meals a day "so that you do not walk around feeling hungry." It also "allows you a morning or afternoon pickup, depending on when you feel fagged out." Also there is an "evening snack" or "night cap" to be taken before going to bed "to prevent 'night hunger'."

But the statement about this phoney reducing program, that contains plenty of "health food" products, that I want to discuss is the following:

"Besides permitting you these liberties, the Dipsy Diet insists on a fairly generous breakfast. Most diets allow very little for breakfast. This does not seem very sensible when one considers the fact that an entire night has gone by without food, and a full day is just ahead of you. The Dipsy Diet refuels you at the time that you need your energy foods most. It demands that you eat a good breakfast to give enough energy to start the day."

How much "energy" does one derive from his breakfast with which to start his day? None. The breakfasts given in the menus in the "health food" almanac require three and a half to four hours to complete stomach digestion. When they pass into the intestine they require several more hours for digestion to be completed.

This fallacy that one gets "energy" from food while it is still in the stomach and intestine being digested and before it has reached the cells by way of the blood was fully exposed by Dr. Dewey in various of his writings and in one still obtainable, entitled *The No-Breakfast Plan and Fasting Cure.*

Only the man who is ignorant of physiology can seriously think that breakfast supplies energy with which to start the day. For, even under the best of conditions, it does not reach the blood until hours later.

The food energy with which we start the day is derived from the food eaten the day before, or the week before, or the month before. There are always food stores in the body that are available for instant use if one misses one or several meals.

There is comparatively little energy expenditure during a night of repose. "Sweet, restful sleep," reiterated Dewey, "is not a hunger producer." On the contrary, the night of rest and sleep is the preparation for the next day of activity and one can't sit up all night and consume plenty of "energy foods" and prepare himself for the next day's work.

Completion of the work of digestion of the food eaten the day before and the evening before is made during the night and it is carried to the liver and other storage places and to the cells and, by morning, is ready to supply the working energy for the day.

It is wrong to think that because no food has been eaten since six o'clock the evening before, therefore, no food has been finding its way into the blood and from here to the cells during the night. It is folly to imagine the food eaten the preceding evening has all been used up in work during the night so that there is no "food energy" with which to start the day unless a liberal breakfast is eaten.

There is not even good evidence that when food is completely digested and absorbed, it is immediately available for use in work. There are reasons for believing some of it, at least; must undergo further changes and modifications before it is ready for use by the cells. The amino acids are known to undergo changes as they are picked up by the walls of the intestines and secreted into the blood stream.

Men who can seriously refer to eating as "refueling" and who have the old fire-box conception of nutrition may well overlook the facts of physiology, even if they know them, and write their sales articles in a way to sell their worthless wares. I would not take up space to expose these fallacies that issue in a flood from the "health food" industry if it were not for the fact that so many thousands of people think these "health food" salesmen and storekeepers know what they are talking about and go to them for dietetic advice.

Reversing the above argument, the "health food" almanac continues: "In the middle of the day the amount of food in the Dipsy Diet goes down, compared with usual diets. This fact is important when you realize that a large lunch very often gives a person a sluggish, tired feeling. This definitely prevents many people from carrying on their work efficiently and actively in the afternoon."

Does this "sluggish, tired feeling" and the

resulting inefficiency and inactivity come from an overdose of energy? If eating provides immediate energy, why should the midday meal not give the worker a "pick-up"? If a morning or afternoon "pick-up" gives energy, why does the mid-day meal slow one down?

The answer to these questions is quite simple and has been before the world a long time. Intelligent people have made good use of the answer; others have followed the advice of those who sell foods and want you to have "plenty of good nourishing food to keep up your strength." Well or sick, fat or lean, hungry or not, you must eat "plenty of good nourishing food."

All meals, whether light or heavy, whether taken morning, noon or night, or between these times, cause blood and nerve energy to be determined to the digestive organs and away from the brain and muscles. Instead of yielding up energy immediately, energy already possessed is immediately used up in the work of digesting the food.

Digestion is most efficient when body, mind and emotions are at rest. It is less efficient as physical, mental and emotional activities mount. We either work hard and retard or suspend digestion, or we work lightly or not at all and permit digestion to proceed smoothly. A hearty breakfast can and does produce just as much sluggishness and inefficiency as a hearty noon meal.

The ideal time for the heavy meal of the day is after the day's work is done when there is leisure time for digestion. But this certainly should not be poured in upon two previous meals of the same day, which, due to work, have not been digested. Intelligent men and women have learned this fact and either eat no breakfast at all or eat but a light breakfast and a light lunch. Dr. Dewey amply proved both with farmers and office workers that the omission of breakfast resulted in increased vigor and efficiency. Graham seems to have been the first modern advocate of the two meals a day plan, but Dewey made a major issue of it.

I have tried both the two-meals-a-day and the one-meal-a-day plans for long periods and found them better than three meals a day. But neither of these plans is ideal. Dewey emphasized the practice of eating only when hungry. This is the ideal and if carried out, it would do away with all plans of eating a particular number of meals each day and with the practice of having meals at regular times each day. It is simply difficult for most men and women to carry out under working conditions.

Fasting Vindicated

Did you see that brief account of an experiment conducted by the Army Air Forces in the Gulf of Mexico to determine the problem of survival at sea, carried in Nov. 2, issue of *Look?* Men were put out in life-rafts and remained there several days under all the weather conditions they are likely to encounter in case of being forced down at sea.

These men were taken aboard ship a few minutes each day for examinations and tests. One 38 year old officer went without food and water for four days, refraining from smoking during this period. He is said to have "felt no ill effects." The account adds: "Others on short rations, suffered more."

The fact that the faster suffered less than those who were on short rations will surprise no one experienced with fasting. Upton Sinclair, Prof. Morgullis, the present writer and many others have repeatedly called attention to this fact. Many times it has been demonstrated that an animal will be killed much quicker by a diet of white bread, or white sugar, or meat soup and similar diets, than by abstinence from all food. This fact does not hold true for long periods of abstinence from water.

It is not enough, however, to find that when a fit man goes without food for four days, he suffers no ill effects. Fasting results in positive benefits and these seem to have been overlooked in making this test. We turn, then, to another source for the testimony of an enemy of fasting to show that it does produce positive bene-

fits. The man we quote below has more than
once condemned fasting in his published articles. The fact that he now offers his approval
of fasts of short duration, is significant.

In his syndicated article of October 23, Irving
S. Cutter, M. D., discusses "Fasting — an Aid in
Lowering Blood-pressure." He offers the suggestion that fasting is a "long discarded healing
procedure." It is true that it is a very old procedure, but it was never discarded by nature,
and there has never been a time when it was not
used even by man. But to return to Cutter's article, he says:

The other evening, reading over the cases of
one of the wisest of our physicians, I was struck
by his frequent use of fasting in the treatment
of hardening of the arteries, diabetes, gout and
other kidney disease. Many cures were reported
and several of his patients were followed for years.

During the interval, some took nothing but
water, while others were allowed fruits and fruit-
juices. In fact, where a two-to-five-day bout was
in prospect, he would permit the rather free use
of orange juice for the first day, ultimately limit-
ing the diet to weak tea.

We cannot fail to recognize the common sense
which dictates the plan. Most of us ingest too
much food, and the constant overfilling of the
alimentary tract actually clogs the flues of digestion, interferes with oxidation, and thus over-
loads the organs of elimination. Appetite can become akin to drug-addiction, demanding edibles
for satisfaction—a full stomach. This must have
been the case with that valiant trencherman,
"Diamond Jim" Brady.

A fruit diet is not a fast and we must not
overlook the fact that all the cases recorded by
this wise physician were not fasting cases. On
the other hand, the fruit diet or fruit juice diet,
if not consumed in large quantities, produces

many of the results effected by the fast. The use of tea, however weak, is to be condemned.

Food-addiction, or food-drunkenness, is an old story in Hygienic literature. This is the first mention I have seen of it in "regular" medical literature. I fear to hope that its recognition spells progress.

"How long can starvation continue?" asks Cutter. The question is "irrelevant' immaterial and inconsequential." He is not discussing starving, but fasting, and he should learn the distinction between the two processes. Cutter answers his question in the following words:

One day a week for the person of normal weight can be endured without the slightest harm. Two days a month may be experienced with ease. But for the individual with high blood-pressure, a week every two or three months may lower the pound within the arteries to a satisfactory level.

Fasting one day a week is a very old practice as references to the custom in the Bible show. Fasting two days a month is also an old practice. Fasting a week every two or three months is by no means new. But short fasts of this nature are seldom enough to accomplish any marked improvements in one who is really sick. Nor do such short periods of abstinence answer the question: "How long can starvation (fasting) continue?"

Cutter actually discovers that nature takes away the desire for food in "infection." He says:

Mild starvation for a short time is a valuable remedy which may be adopted with profit by many. It is exactly the thing which nature takes whenever an infection takes away the desire for food. Of course, it cannot be applied to those who are undernourished or who exhibit a blood-pressure which is quite too low.

Cutter has had no experience with fasting. If the advice he gives for conducting a fast is borrowed from the wise physician whose cases he read over, we cannot think too highly of his wisdom. Let Cutter tell us how to conduct the fast. He says:

If the management is inaugurated, no laxatives will be required. Generous quantities of water will assist the body in getting rid of toxins. Furthermore the skin will increase its activity. One of the chief complaints during the process is that the body seems to emit a foul odor. This is ample proof that undesirable products are departing.

Under a carefully supervised program, more often than not the blood-pressure will fall. If it goes below 110 systolic, some food or activity may be demanded, but for the one who has been accustomed to a reading of 180 or even higher, the drop should be gradual. As poisons are excreted, there will be notable return of energy. There is no need to remain in bed, although periods of rest may alternate with short walks.

For the first 24 to 48 hours, headache may be encountered. Hot water or weak tea is the answer. The urine should be watched for the apperance of acidosis, in which event small amounts of bicarbonate of soda may be given. Hunger pains will also be mentioned, but will rarely persist if orange-juice is administered.

No laxative is required — this is correct. Our experience has shown that in fasting there will be bowel movement when there is need for one and that it is safe to wait if the bowels do not act.

There is no need for the "generous quantities of water" and drinking water in large quantities will not assist the body in getting rid of toxins— the body only gets rid of the excess of water at some cost to itself. Drink only when thirsty.

Skin activity is increased during the fast. Elimination is increased during the fast. Blood-pressure will fall but there is no need for food or activity because blood-pressure falls below 110.

The excretion of toxins is followed by increased energy. Increase of strength often results from fasting, even fasts of considerable length, often result in increase of strength.

There is no need to remain in bed for a fast of two days. But if one is sick and needs a lengthy fast, it is best to go to bed and conserve the energies and resources of the body. The ship-wrecked man on the life raft could last longer without food, if circumstances did not force a rapid expenditure of his internal resources.

Hot water and weak tea are not to be used to relieve headache. This belongs to the "doctoring" habit. Tea will be avoided at all times by intelligent men and women.

Watching the urine for the "appearance of acidosis" is a foolish procedure. Fasting does not produce acidosis. It has the contrary effect.

Neither soda nor any other drug should be given during a fast. To give soda to "relieve" acidosis is an old medical practice and does not belong to fasting.

There are no such things as hunger-pains, though there are often discomforts in the stomach region, but orange juice need not be given to "relieve" these. The really healthy person experiences no discomfort when fasting. The sick person presents a variety of reactions. There need be no fear of them.

After the reader has perused the above let him not excite himself with the thought that the medical profession is on the verge of adopting fasting as a part of their practice. If an occasional medical man adopts fasting, as an occasional one does diet, it does not mean that the profession will do so — at least, not for some time. Why should they resort to fasting while they have sulfa-drugs and penicillin?

Growing Old

In one of his recent newspaper "Let's Explore Your Mind" items, Albert Edward Wiggam, D.Sc., asks:

"Can you tell a person's age by counting the candles on his birthday cake?"

He answers as follows:

"Not by from 10 to 25 years. As Marjorie Greenbie points out in her book that I like immensly, 'Be Your Age,' a man who has lived fast and hard and worn out his heart and endocrine glands may really be 70 whereas Dr. Wingate Todd shows in the Scientific Monthly a man of 60 or 70 who has lived on a proper diet — may have all the alertness, grace and charm, and both the mental and physical age of a man of 40 or 50. As the new psychology and discoveries in nutrition prove, it is not only nonsense but downright ignorance, nowadays, to classify people's ages by their birthdays."

It has taken a long time for men and women like Wiggam, Greenbie and Todd to make even the little progress the above quotation indicates. Outside the ranks of the "scientific thinkers" it has been heralded for years that a man may be old at forty or young at eighty. The discoveries in nutrition which Wiggam refers to were made long ago outside the ranks of "regular" medicine and "regular" science. It is difficult to decide just what the "new psychology" has to do with the discoveries he so belatedly acknowledges.

The "scientists" tell us that there are three kinds of ages — *Chronological age* which represents the number of years we have lived; *Physio-*

logical age which represents the stage of physical development we have achieved; *Psychological age* which represents the stage of mental development we have reached.

Now, since physiological development reaches its end sometime between the twentieth and thirtieth years of life, it should be obvious that the term *Physiological age* is not properly applied to the later years of life.

Since the aging process, by which I mean the changes in the body that we call "old age", is a pathological process, a gradual deterioration of the body, we should use the term *Pathological age* to designate the stage of physical wreckage we have reached.

Physical wreckage is not measured in years but by the amount of damage that has resulted to the organs and functions of the body. This damage is determined by the kind of life we live.

Bear in mind that "old age" is not merely "worn out heart and endocrine glands." All of the organs and tissues are involved — the muscles, nerves, digestive organs, liver, kidneys, skin, etc.

The phrase, "lived fast and hard" is not very definite. It is susceptible of varied interpretations. In this instance its meaning is probably as empty as Dr. Todd's "proper diet." The doctor probably knows very little about what constitutes a proper diet and Miss Greenbie probably makes numerous compromises with wrong living.

Human life is lived on a haphazzard, a hit-or-miss plan, often without even an element of suggestion of the precautions employed in running the simplest kind of business or in caring for a simple piece of machinery. Even a peanut vendor exercises more system in running his stand than the average "educated" man or woman uses in his business of living.

The trend in diet today is to eat something from each of the "basic seven" groups of foods. In other words, the government, the pseudo-dietitians and the food manufacturers have gotten together and devised a scheme to encourage the people to eat everything the manufacturers offer and to give no heed to the voices of the reformers. As the "basic seven" plan of eating has the endorsement of the drugging profession and of the "scientists," there can be no doubt that Dr. Todd and Miss Greenbie recommend it in their books.

Old age is a disease and hence, theoretically and practically, to a marked degree, at least, avoidable on a new way of living and thinking. A large part of our way of living is crudely inept and is not even consistent with a pleasurable and happy existence.

What we term old age (or aging) is a state of actual organic disease which has not yet advanced far enough to prevent the organs from performing their functions, although these functions are crippled. Disease is preventable—aging is preventable. We should seek emancipation from, rather than resignation to, old age. But on every hand today, we see, on one side, a needless fear of disease and, on the other side, a stupid neglect of the early signs of disease.

We could if we would, not only avoid much of the aging process, but we could also greatly extend our life-span. We are not hurried to the grave by a ridiculous old man with a scythe and an hour glass, but by the breakdown of vital organs so that they can no longer perform their duties.

This breakdown of organs is the result of acute and chronic poisoning (toxemia) and the stresses we habitually place upon them by our chaotic living. It is only man's ignorance of and ignoring of the factors of causation that so affect his body in the course of time that prevents him from effecting a very substantial extension of his life span.

Organs are not fated, as is taught in some quarters, to break down at certain times of life. When they succumb depends upon how much they are stressed by an enervating mode of living and the resulting toxemia. That organs are not fated to break down at the times stated is shown by the fact that only relatively small percentages of them in the population as a whole, actually do break down at the times they are said to be fated to break. And in these cases, poisoning, not fate, accounts for their collapse.

Fate has no place in biology and physiology and is not an etiological factor in pathology. Nor is time, *per se*, a cause of disease or aging. Aging takes place in time, but is not caused by time. It is the cumulative effect of many impairing influences that operate in time or over a period of time. We have it in our own hands to largely determine how much and how soon we age.

Diseases of Middle Age

I believe it was Pope who advised:
"Presume not God to scan
The proper study of Mankind is Man."
Quarles says: "Man is man's A. B. C. There is none that can read God aright, unless he first spell man."

A study of man is one of the most vital needs of today. For ages our wise men studied the gods, the devils, the stars and all things other than Man in their efforts to understand Man. From these studies we have inherited a vast storehouse of useless lore that is very much in our way.

During the past hundred years, or nearly so, our wise men have trained their microscopes upon bacteria and protozoa and have dissected and vivisected untold millions of rats, mice, cats, dogs, guinea pigs, monkeys and other animals and even plants in their endeavor to understand man. The biologist studies the corpse of animals, the psychologist observes the behavior of grass-hoppers, in an endeavor to understand man. Nobody studies Man. It is the medical view that the proper study of mankind is rats.

We have a group of wise men who are c a l l e d anthropologists. Anthropology is the *Science of Man.* To these men, then, we should look for knowledge of man. We should expect to find them engaged in the study of Man.

But if we turn to these men we are again disappointed. They do not study Man. Instead they dig around among the pieces of broken pottery and the crumbled ruins of once thriving cities and delve into the superstitions of "savages" and write learned tomes about these grave yards. Much of their assumed knowledge of the past is pure guess work. They do not study, they have not studied, Man.

"The proper study of mankind is Man," but man is as unknown today as he was a few years ago when Carrel wrote his book — *Man The Unknown.* "Man is Man's A. B. C.," but there are so few who can even begin to read him.

How few know the signs of health! How many know from experience the signs of disease! Yet, are there a hundred men in the world who can distinguish a healthy from an unhealthy man? Do we not daily see the obviously sick person passed as healthy?

What is *disease?* What is the relation of man's habits to the development of his *disease?* What effect will a change of habits have upon his health? These questions are foolishness unto the average physician.

What is a cold? Everybody assumes that he knows what a cold is. Research specialists of all kinds have searched and researched, singly and in combinations, times without number, for the cause of *colds.* Always their efforts end in failure.

They do not know what a cold is. They do not know the cause of colds. They have no *cure* for colds. They do not know how to prevent colds. Cold *cures* by the millions have been tried — and found wanting. Cold *preventives* galore have been employed — all without success.

The cold is the first "organized" pathology. It is one of the simplest forms of "disease." It represents the early beginning of the many complex and compound pathologies to which hundreds of confusing names have been given.

The physician who does not understand this simple pathology, does not know its cause, but who presumes to understand the more complex later stages of pathology is living in a fool's paradise.

A cold is the beginning, the *alpha*, of a pathological chain of which cancer may be the ending, the *omega*. A profession that seeks for a *cure* for cancer and assures us that it is right now standing on the threshold of that discovery, yet acknowledges that it knows nothing of the beginning of the development of the pathological evolution of which cancer is the end-point, is merely stupid. How can they expect to prevent or *cure* a compound pathology, such as cancer, when they can neither prevent nor *cure* a cold?

Medical nomenclature is a meaningless jargon. It has hundreds of names for various pathological stages and variations, fundamental understanding of which is lacking.

Tilden says: "The most advanced medical thought of today is a tangled web — a little distorted truth in both woof and warp of the so-called science, but without system or order — order, the first law of heaven." All medical practice is a slap in the face of law and order. It is an effort to cure disease without removing cause. It seeks to prevent cancer without knowing the cause of cancer. It refuses to recognize cancer as an end-point in a pathological evolution that had its beginning in infancy. It seeks to cure arthritis without knowing its cause.

The first signs of arthritis (the first symptoms of any evolving pathology) may and commonly do appear years before the particular symptom-complex that has received the name of *arthritis* is established. Even the first recognized signs of arthritis often put in their appearance years before *arthritis* becomes established. If, at this stage ,the manner of living is corrected, further evolution, even of heart complications, will be prevented.

People who develop kidney disease have abused themselves all their lives. They have poisoned themselves with tobacco, alcohol and gastro-intestinal decomposition until their kidneys could stand it no longer. They have lived haphazardly until chronic disease is fully established and they become pessimistic because a profession that insists on treating each phase of the evolution of *disease*, as a separate *disease*, can offer them no hope.

"The babe catches cold," says Tilden; "at eighty it dies of high blood pressure, hard arteries, heart disease, rheumatism,etc. etc." These are each and all evolutional results of a mode of living that does violence to all the vital interests of life. The cold was merely the first sign of an established toxemia.

These end-points in pathological evolution are reached years after the first symptoms of constitutional catarrh — colds, sinus "infection," gastritis, colitis, leucorrhea, metritis, etc. — and symptoms of genito-urinary impairment are developed.

The cold is not the real beginning of "disease" — pathology. The foundation for cancer, Bright's disease, diabetes, hardening of the arteries, disease of the heart, nervous disease, arthritis, or any other so-called disease is laid the first day any disease producing habit is started — any physical or mental habit that produces enervation and perversion of nutrition.

"Middle life is a late period," says Tilden "to begin to look for the first signs of any so-called chronic disease." We need to understand that chronic disease begins early — in small, even imperceptible, beginnings. Frequent colds, periods of not feeling well, occasional periods of indigestion, constipation, occasional diarrhea, slight twinges of pain here and there — these are early signs of the development that ends later in the so-called *degenerative diseases of later life*.

Specialists write text-books on "diseases of middle life" — so common are the affections. They describe in great detail their symptoms, variations, complications and endings. They go to great lengths in detailing the "special treatments" of these "middle-age diseases." But these books and their descriptions and treatments do not enable physicians to *cure* these *diseases*.

The treatments are all palliative and suppressive. They do not remove causes. They often remove organs or parts of organs, but they do not correct the life of the patient. Cause is, admittedly, unknown. The early beginnings of these *"diseases"* are unrecognized. The evolution of these various pathologies is not understood. In the midst of so much ignorance the *shaman* offers us nothing but his magic.

When we understand man — when we know his needs and his limitations — we can point the way to life. Today, unfortunately, the hand of the disease trades (the various kinds of schools of "healing") points to death — a premature death preceded by much weakness and suffering.

The "diseases of middle age" are evolutions out of chronic toxemia. Toxemia grows out of chronic abuse of the body. It cannot be too often repeated that chronic disease represents chronic provocation. The care of the body that will prevent colds will prevent the development of the middle age "diseases." Recovery from these "diseases" can occur only when their causes have been removed. The patchwork methods of treatment now in vogue are futile. However much palliation and temporary respite from discomfort these may afford, they are powerless to produce lasting desirable results. Only a reformed life can give lasting results.

Living to Live

In those ancient Hebrew writings that are collectively known to us as the *Old Testament* there is expressed a conception of the way in which *punishment* for "sin" is brought about, that I think we would do well to understand. This *punishment* is described as "even the fruit of their own thoughts."

That *punishment* of wrong doing is not a punishment at all, but a result, a consequence, a fruit of the wrong doing, in other words, a development, is a principle that we need to learn. When we fully understand this principle, we will realize that there is, and can be no vicarious atonement for our "transgression of the law."

Every act and every emotion has its consequence. The act and the consequence are inseparable — as inseparable as light and shadow. *It is, therefore, not possible to do a thing without setting in motion the necessary train of consequences — of reactions.*

This same principle is well expressed in the statement that "we are punished by our sins, not for them." No third thing punishes us for sticking our hand in the fire. We are *punished* by putting our hand in the fire. The burning of our hand is the consequence of putting it into the fire — it is the fruit of the act. The result of every act is inherent in and concurrent with the act. *Every wrong action sets in motion the necessary train of bad consequences — of bad reactions.* This being true, we cannot escape the full consequence of whatever we do.

Fortunately natural laws work both ways. *Rewards* for virtues may, with equal correctness be described as "even the fruit of their own thoughts". We are *rewarded* by our virtues, not for them. Every right act has good consequences, just as surely as every wrong act has bad consequences. *Every right action sets in motion the necessary train of good consequences — of good reactions.* This being true we cannot be robbed of the full consequence of whatever we do.

Good health is "even the fruit of their own thoughts" and actions, just as poor health (disease) is "even the fruit of their own thoughts" and actions. Gluttony produces evil consequences, moderation produces good consequences. Drunkenness sets in motion a whole train of bad reactions, abstinence does not produce these bad reactions.

There is no "beyond good and evil." Evil is that which has harmful consequences. Good is that which has helpful consequences. Evil is that which detracts from the powers of life and tends towards death. Good is that which enhances the powers of life and avails towards greater life. Here is the measure of *right* and *wrong*. Here is the criterion by which any mode of living is to be judged.

That is right living which produces and maintains health and happiness and increases life. That is wrong living which impairs health, produces misery and decreases life.

To be more specific, right living is that living which conforms in all of its details with the laws of life; wrong living is that living that in part or much of its details is in conflict with these laws.

The laws of life are not something imposed upon the organization of man. They are imbedded in the very structure of our being, in our tissues, our nerve and muscle cells, our blood-stream, into the total organism. They are the way we are constituted to live. If we live according to them, we live; if we do not live according to them, we don't truly live. Since these laws are fundamental parts of us we cannot revolt against them without revolting against ourselves. They are the fountain of life and when we flout them we cease to drink at that fountain.

Natural law represents the way things are made to work. If you try to work some other way you work your own ruin. Wrong living is an effort to live against the very nature of things; it is an endeavor to flout the very constitution of being, to divorce oneself from that fundament upon which life rests, and it ends only in destruction. The wrong liver renders himself unfit to survive. He breaks down, disintegrates, perishes. He refuses to observe the laws of life, so he rots and is no more.

We cannot run away from the laws of being without running away from ourselves. There simply is no escape, except in death. The sum-total of the modern revolt against nature is this: *we who have decided we cannot and will not live with nature soon come to find that we cannot live with ourselves.* The man who flouts the laws of nature is not merely a problem to those around him, he is a problem to himself.

All you have is life and you have this only as you live it. You cannot abuse it with impunity. Your life is constituted to work one way —it will not work any other. Written into the flesh and blood and stamped in the total organization of life are the eternal, immutable and inflexible laws of nature, and no one can break them, although he can break himself in the attempt.

"Evil," it has been said, "is the great illusion — it is the illusion that you can live against the design of nature and get away with it." Wrong living is literally to miss that for which we are inwardly and fundamentally constituted. In its broadest meaning, wrong living is self-abuse. It is an effort to live by wrong principles, and when the principles of life are wrong, all of life goes wrong with them.

Health and disease are not something extraneously given. They are inherent results. They result from opposite modes of living. We cannot do as we please, for some ways are superior to other ways. Only the superior ways produce superior results. Inferior ways destroy those who practice them.

The laws of nature are not only stamped into our very being; they are also stamped into our relationships with the whole of life and of nature. You can violate the laws of relationship but you destroy yourself in doing it. You are related to food, water, air, sunshine, other people, other forms of life, etc. You have one type of relationship to food and another type of relationship to poisons. It behooves you to know and understand these relationships and be guided accordingly.

As an entity, a living self-acting organism, you have a certain choice in the way you live. You exercise autonomy. You can choose to use alcohol or to abstain, to be a vegetarian or to eat flesh, to take exercise or to remain idle, to live in the shadows or out in the sun, to dissipate your sex energies or conserve them, etc. You are free to choose your own way of life, but you are not free to choose the results. The consequences of your choice are "even the fruit of your own thoughts" and actions. We either build ourselves or we destroy ourselves by the manner in which we live.

Life is not a matter of "do this", and "don't do that." It is a matter of relationships. If you get into right relationships everything follows from that. Everything flows from the central loyalty. Health flows from loyalty to the legitimate, disease from loyalty to the illegitimate things of life.

All living is a curious mixture of right and wrong conduct — of good food and bad, of fresh air and foul, of conservation and dissipation, of of temperance in one thing and overindulgence in another. There is, then, a great need for self-discipline in harmony with the laws of being. We need to learn the true principles of life and align our lives with them.

"I have used coffee for twenty years and I am not dead yet." An ancient Hebrew writer provided the answer centuries ago, when he said: "Because sentence against an evil work is not executed speedily it is, therefore, fully written in the heart of man to do evil." You looked for consequences to come as a thunderbolt from the hand of an angry Jove and since you were not struck dead, you think nothing has happened. You deceive yourself. Inner deterioration and decay have set in and have progressed and sooner or later the disintegration will become great enough to force itself upon your attention.

You may never realize that you have destroyed yourself. You may die in your delusion that nothing hurts you, that you can violate all the laws of life with impunity. Sylvester Graham had such as you in mind when he declared that the grand experiment of the whole human race seems ever to have been to ascertain just how far they can go in indulgence without dying so suddenly and violently as to be compelled to know they have destroyed themselves.

If the nature of things guarantees the instability of evil, it also guarantees the stability of good. When you do that which is right the whole universe backs you up; when you do that which is wrong the whole universe is arrayed against you. No amount of cleverness and scheming on the part of physicians can hold wrong living and wrong treatment together. In the end they collapse for the universe is not built for the success of fallacy. Life is not constituted for the triumph of wrong.

If you desire truly to live you will cease trying to find magic tricks and short-cuts to life and learn the simple laws of being and order your life in conformity with these. Realign your life with the laws of nature—this and this alone constitutes *living to live*.

Born an Original —
Died a Copy

Ours is the age of carbon copies, of *cliche* minds and of closest conformity to the customs of the society in which we unfortunately live. Perhaps there was never a time in the past history of civilization when the non-conformist was so rare and so unpopular as he is today in America. The irony of the situation lies in the fact that this condition has arisen at the very time that psychologists are advising, *"be yourself"*, and teachers are urging children to express themselves.

We are all born *originals*; practically all of us die *copies*. Society turns us on its educational lathe and molds us in its stereotyped molds and turns out more or less uniform products. America resembles nothing so much as a huge mass-production plant, with its children "on the line" being painted and polished like Ford cars and turned out with the same uniformity of design and sameness of performance.

How many of us are not slaves to fashion? Do we not usually drink because this is "the proper thing"? We cook our foods in the customary manner, eat the same breakfast foods, buy the same brand of aspirins, submit to the same operations that our neighbors do.

We wear the customary styles in dress, fix our hair in the regular vogues, follow the fads in nail polish or lip stick and raise or lower our skirts as fashion decrees.

We read the same books, and all too often only those books, which are among the "best sellers," buy the popular magzines, hear only the "approved" (guaranteed to be safe) lecturers, and join only the "best" organizations. We think the thoughts that are in fashion, say the things that others around us are saying; attend the same shows that our neighbors go to, and vote for the popular candidate. Even in our speech we use the popular expressions and follow the fashion in slang.

Most of us are afraid to have an unpopular idea and lack the courage of the older generation that slipped out behind the barn and read the forbidden dime novel.

How many of my readers remember the lines of the old hymn of yesteryear:

> "Dare to be a Daniel
> Dare to stand alone?"

These lines have lost all their meaning to the jelly-fish anthropoids of the present. The admirable old quality to which the name, moral courage, was applied has gone glimmering through the things that were. Today, we would rather be popular than right and we no longer feel that "truth and one make a majority."

Do we not hear young men and women saying that they have to smoke to be popular with the crowd? Do we not hear them saying the same thing about drink? And do not the girls say that they are not popular if they refuse to pet and that the boys won't go with them a second time if they refuse coition?

Is this the kind of material out of which to build and with which to maintain a democracy? These people can't stand on their own feet, but must lean upon the unthinking crowd around them for support. They are lacking in that good, old-fashioned quality called *guts* and are also lacking in the power to think.

We do not blame the young folks as much as we do their parents, teachers, and "spiritual" guides. It is a rare mind that retains any of its native power to think after being run through those intellectual canning factories we call educational institutions. Educators are busy knocking the children's brains out and replacing them with the inferior putty of contentment. It takes more courage than most people have, not to be a conformist after having pounded into them for years the fallacy of the so-called psychologists that intelligence is "ability to solve the problem of adjustment to environmental (in this case social) demands" involving "submissiveness" and "responsiveness."

This is merely a "scientific" dress for the old admonition: "When in Rome do as the Romans do." It is the herd instinct asserting its supremacy in human affairs. It is an echo of the age-long effort to force everybody to be like everybody else. It does not allow for individuality, variation or difference. Conform to the follies of the fools around you, or you are "queer," you are "cracked", you are crazy.

In this day of sham democracy, pseudo-advancement and education by propaganda, our people have lost their courage. They are so afraid of being lost out of the social package on the way down town that they follow the crowd, even if, like a herd of stampeding range cattle, they wind up at the bottom of the bluff.

Such a people are ripe for totalitarian doctrines. They are easy dupes of the propaganda for "unity", "solidarity" and other catch-words and shiboleths with which the manipulators of the mob bait their hooks. They are easily carried away with the claims of those who are supposed to know (but don't) that ours is an age of science and that vaccines, serums, anti-toxins, toxoids, etc., are scientific. These people can be

herded like sheep because the process of knocking their brains out started in infancy and the job
is pretty well completed by the time they are
fifteen years old.

Perhaps nothing so accurately measures their
mental status as the manner and extent to which
they are influenced by the lies of the commercial
broadcasts that fill the air morning, noon and
night.

My old friend Bruce Calvert, founder and
for years, editor of the *Open Road* tried for years
to start a movement to "Make the World Safe
For Intelligence." Unfortunately he couldn't find
enough intelligent people to start the movement.

Men and women of courage will think and act
for themselves and will not be cowed by the
scoffs and jeers of the unthinking crowd. They
will not be afraid to turn aside from the beaten
path to explore new fields. No laughter of fools
will deter them from casting off the dead weight
of fashionable methods of slow suicide and
live, thereafter, a life of principle and rectitude.

Many are willing to take a short detour on
the *Hygienic* road to achieve some end after
which the road is forgotten and they return
to the broad highway of convention and false
pleasure. Experience has proven that such a
course leads only to ultimate failure and disappointment, because it rests upon a basic dis-
honesty.

True happiness and success in life cannot be
had upon any basis of compromise with principle. We need to develop a love of principles
and to discard our fear of the views of the mob.
Shakespeare's words are very fitting here:

"If we stand still
In fear our motion will be mocked or carp'd at,
We should take root here where we sit, sit
State statutes only."

Men and women, young and old, of today, are promiscuously drifting down the river of life, merely helping to make up the great confusion. They have, perhaps uncosciously, dedicated their lives to indulgence and vainly imagine they are under some kind of heavenly compulsion to destroy themselves.

Their's is a rather arrogant view, claiming compulsion too high for their perverted instincts, as though those instincts (or rather those pervertions) were in communion with the solemn majesties of Nature, which they are not. As a result of men's indulgencies, they have become diseased and they have developed the fatalistic idea that they have to suffer, that disease is a kind of *ineluctable fatum*, which they hardly wish to defy if they can, and hardly can if they desire.

Those who desire to be entirely unshackled, as though uncontrolled easiness of life can give them all they require, should know that such living easily leads to an uncontrolled appetite and a plethoric condition of body, which in the end prove fatal.

Fasting Versus Dieting

John W. Armstrong of England has had a wide experience with fasting and diets. A few years ago one of his patients fasted 101 days and recovered from total blindness during the fast. I believe he puts his finger on a sore spot when he says that "the reason fasting is not more popular amongst practitioners is because few of them know much about it and have, therefore, neither the knowledge, experience or faith to present it to their patients." He calls fasting "the oldest and sanest practice of all time in the treatment of most diseases." Hygienists do not regard fasting as a treatment of disease, but otherwise the fact stated by Armstrong is acceptable.

Recently a woman came to the Health School from St. Louis. She had a lengthy fast while here. For some time before coming to the health school she had trouble with her finger nails and was assured by the health food authorities to whom she went that her troubles were due to calcium deficiency. She faithfully swallowed the calcium preparations supplied by the health food store and also took other food preparations with which they supplied her. For some time she followed the advice given by these food experts, but her nail condition did not improve. On the contrary, it grew worse.

During the fast the nail condition completely recovered. When she left the Health School all traces of her former nail condition had disappeared. Now, fasting does not supply calcium to the body. We give our fasting guests distilled water to drink and there is no calcium in this. The health food stores are talking "deficiency" to the people all over the country and the so-called health lecturers are talking "deficiency" and both the lecturers and the stores are selling all manners of preparations to make good the "deficiencies." And all over America there are millions of people who are living testimonials to the fallacy of the theory and the practice.

Armstrong says "there have been fasting failures." I do not agree with this statement. Fasting is not a cure and if one does not get well while fasting it does not mean that fasting is a failure. Fasting never fails to accomplish its one and only purpose—that of giving the functions of the body an opportunity to rest. That the body sometimes fails to heal itself during even a prolonged fast is true, but it is only true in cases that have reached the irremediable stage or in cases in which the patient cannot fast long enough at one time to secure results. This does not mean that fasting failed, however. The fasting gave the needed opportunity for rest, even in these cases.

Attempting to account for some of these "failures" Armstrong says: "if my experience counts for anything, I should say a great error has been made in confusing the *fruit-juice diet* with the *cold-water fast*." Referring to one of his own experiences, he tells of being fasted during four months, in 1916-17, under the care of a "medical convert to the fasting cure" for diabetes, chest trouble, pericarditis and stasis. He says: "His method was "four days in each week on cold water and the remaining three days of each seven a diet he called 'eliminating.'

"I found the diet more weakening and far more irritating than the cold-water days of the fast ever were. After sixteen weeks of it he was in despair and had no answer when I called his method 'the cat and mouse act', and began a real fast on my own responsibility. I fasted forty-seven days without a break and cured the lot —diabetes, chest trouble, pericarditis and stasis."

He says of appendicitis (and what passes for it "urgently needing" surgical intereference), flu, pneumonia, anemia, dropsy, diphtheria, malaria, pruritis, psoriasis, conjunctivitis and ordinary rheumatism, "I personally know people who were restored to normal in each and all of these diseases by the intelligent application of the cold water fasting cure * * * And I do not lose sight of the fact that most of them were not responding favorably to any one of the various reformed diets."

In my own work I have cared for hundreds, even thousands, of people who have been on one or more of the various diets prescribed by various dietitians and pratitioners and who have failed to recover while on these diets. It would not be true to say that none of them had ever made any improvement on some of these diets, but it would be true to say that many of them had continued to grow worse on the diets. A great percentage of these people have made their first improvement while fasting. When years of dieting fail to restore health it is a common experience to get well in a few weeks of fasting.

Armstrong mentions A. Rabagliati, M.D., F.R.C.S., F.R.C.P., Major R.F.E. Austin, M.R.-C.S., L.R.C.P., Dr. H. M. Shelton, Dr. J. H. Tilden, Dr. Arthur Ves, who he says: "all speak very highly of fasting." "Yet all of these," he says, "are world-renowned authorities on dietetics." He thinks that since these men are authorities on dietetics, yet employ and recommend fasting so extensively, fasting accomplishes a work that diet does not and cannot do.

Dr. Rabagliati frequently remarked that the most popular criticisms of fasting and dietetics are written by people who have niether missed a meal in their lives nor done more than *read* half-a-dozen books on reformed dietetics. Out of the depth of their ignorance and inexperience these peole give the world liberal supplies of their great stores of wisdom.

An amazing phenomenon of the present is the steady stream of people into the health food stores of the country in search of adivce about eating and diet cures for their ills. Here are a lot of clerks and grocerymen who have a store house full of wares to sell and who have little knowledge of the human body, or its requirements, of its ills, and of the care it needs, handing out advice to the people who come into the store and selling the various packaged remedies they have on their shelves. Recently I was in a health food store run by a woman whom I have known since she was a little girl. I know that she has never had any training that would in any way equip her to advise the sick. A woman was in the store and had told the health food store proprietor her troubles. The health food store owner sold her a box of synthetic vitamins, a pluri-vitamin product containing all the vitamins, with the explanation that these vitamins would enable her to assimilate whatever was lacking in her system. She did not know what was wrong with the woman, but she had a shotgun prescription that was good for whatever ailed her.

I need not emphasize the fact that the woman got no benefit from taking the pills. She was enervated and toxemic for which there were dozens of causes in her daily life and the pills would not correct a single one of these many causes. A fast would have enabled her body to speed its processes of elimination, a rest would have enabled her to recuperate her nervous energy. But only a complete correction of her mode of living could enable her to make full recovery. No pill, no matter what its nature and composition, can ever substitute for first class habits.

"Many fasts for chronic disease fail for just one thing," says Armstrong, "the patient puts a time limit on the adventure before he starts, and many more break the fast just as soon as their well-meaning, but ill-advised or ill-informed, friends put 'the wind up' the would-be emulator of Matthew iv. 3, 4." He again quates the bible, saying, "He that endureth to the end shall be saved."

Armstrong further says: "Most people think a fast of ten days or less should be sufficient to clear up any disease; and in fasting say a fifth of the time that should be done for half the cases where fasting is indicated, merely stir up mud that does not settle peaceably when feeding is too quickly (and often wrongfully) resumed and are easily led to believe that the penance has harmed them. On top of this the average fruit-juice 'fast' is a farce—in a number of well-seated or 'chronic' disease a mere irritant, and really a very one-sided diet." He mentions Edgar J. Saxon, another British authority on fasting and dietetics, as concurring in this view. Saxon is a man of wide experience.

In 1936 Armstrong wrote: "I have seen over 3,000 people fast in my way since 1918, many of them for quite serious disease after trying divers other means. The longest fasts I have seen were fasts of 90, 93, and 101 days. Fasts of 30 to 40 days have been quite common."

Jennings employed the long fast, as did Page, Walter, Dewey, Tanner, Rabagliati, Kieth, Haddon, Austin, Tilden, Weger, Vos, Hazzard and many others. My own experience has convinced me that in the great majority of cases a long fast is needed; also that one long fast is far more satisfactory than a series of short fasts. Carrington came to the conclusion from his studies and observations of fasting that it is injurious to break a fast before the return of hunger. Although it is not possible in all cases to carry the fast to this point, there is merit in Carrington's veiw.

When these men and women speak of fasting they mean complete abstinence from all food except water. When they place a patient on a fast they give no food but water. They do not call a fruit diet, or a fruit juice diet a fast. I have employed fruit diets and fruit juice diets as have most or all of these people, but our experience has shown us that in those cases where a fast is needed only a fast will serve. Tilden pointed out that the benefits derived from the juice diet are due to the fact that it represents a reduction of food and not to any deficiency the juices are supposed to fill. He pointed out that the less juice taken (this is to say, the nearer to a complete fast one approaches) the greater are the benefits of the juice diet, whereas, if it supplied deficient elements, this would not be so. There is a time factor involved also. A fast will enable the body to accomplish in a short time what it will accomplish on juice only in a much longer period, although there are benefits from fasting that seem never to result from the juice diets.

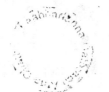